Quest for the Cure

Quest for the Cure

Reflections on the Evolution of Breast Cancer Treatment

George R. Blumenschein, MD

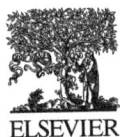

ELSEVIER

AMSTERDAM • BOSTON • HEIDELBERG • LONDON
NEW YORK • OXFORD • PARIS • SAN DIEGO
SAN FRANCISCO • SINGAPORE • SYDNEY • TOKYO
Academic Press is an imprint of Elsevier

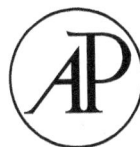

Academic Press is an imprint of Elsevier
The Boulevard, Langford Lane, Kidlington, Oxford, OX5 1GB, UK
225 Wyman Street, Waltham, MA 02451, USA

First published 2014

Notices

Knowledge and best practice in this field are constantly changing. As new research and experience broaden our understanding, changes in research methods, professional practices, or medical treatment may become necessary.

Practitioners and researchers must always rely on their own experience and knowledge in evaluating and using any information, methods, compounds, or experiments described herein. In using such information or methods they should be mindful of their own safety and the safety of others, including parties for whom they have a professional responsibility.

To the fullest extent of the law, neither the Publisher nor the authors, contributors, or editors, assume any liability for any injury and/or damage to persons or property as a matter of products liability, negligence or otherwise, or from any use or operation of any methods, products, instructions, or ideas contained in the material herein.

British Library Cataloguing-in-Publication Data
A catalogue record for this book is available from the British Library

Library of Congress Cataloging-in-Publication Data
A catalog record for this book is available from the Library of Congress

ISBN: 978-0-12-420153-8

For information on all Academic Press publications
visit our website at store.elsevier.com

This book has been manufactured using Print On Demand technology. Each copy is produced to order and is limited to black ink. The online version of this book will show color figures where appropriate.

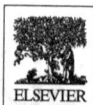

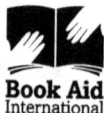

CONTENTS

ACKNOWLEDGMENTS

First of all, I would like to thank and dedicate this book to the patients whose confidence provided me with the strength and motivation to persist in the quest for a cure for breast cancer. I am also indebted to Patty Decker, my physician's assistant, and to nurses Kim Wagner, Shelley Dodd, and Melissa Hach who provided outstanding care for my patients and, together with Kathy White, my administrative assistant, encouraged me to write this book. Joni Rodgers provided invaluable help in moving the project ahead and in providing the foreword for this book. My medical school classmate, Arthur J. Atkinson, Jr., provided subsequent editing and technical assistance. The staff at Elsevier were essential to making successful production of the book a reality and were a pleasure to work with. Finally, this book would never have been written without the unflagging support of my wife, Sarah Deitrick Blumenschein, MD, for which I shall be eternally grateful.

FOREWORD

In 2008, I was hired to coauthor a memoir with Ambassador Nancy Brinker, founder of Susan G. Komen for the Cure. (*Promise Me: How a Sister's Love Launched the Global Movement to End Breast Cancer* was published by Random House in 2010.)

"You need to talk to Blumenschein," she told me at our very first meeting. "He's important."

Dr. George Blumenschein was the oncologist who'd treated Nan's sister Suzy in the last year of her life. Suzy had been diagnosed with breast cancer in 1977, and Nancy believes that if Suzy had gone to Dr. Blumenschein initially, it's possible that Suzy would be alive today. As fate would have it, Suzy was treated by a surgeon who performed a lumpectomy and came out of the operating room to tell Suzy's family, "I got it all. She's cured."

Less than a year later, Suzy called her sister in a panic. There was a lump under her arm. Nancy, who worked in marketing at Neiman Marcus in Dallas, had done a lot of fundraising for various charities, including the American Cancer Society. She called in all her connections, asking, "Who's the absolute best?" She was told to take Suzy to Dr. George Blumenschein at the M.D. Anderson Cancer Center in Houston. After a failed course of radiation treatment at Mayo Clinic, Suzy agreed to come to Texas.

In *Promise Me*, Nancy describes Dr. Blumenschein as "indisputably in charge," a Yale man who'd gone on to medical school at Cornell and postgraduate work at Bellevue Hospital in New York, the National Cancer Institute in Bethesda, MD, and Duke University Hospital in North Carolina.

"His credentials were varied and impressive," she writes, "his work was well known and respected, and his patients adored him for his gentle good humor. I remember being awed by Dr. Blumenschein's breadth of knowledge and so very grateful for the way he empowered Suzy with hard information and encouraged her with realistic hope."

Suzy (being inimitably Suzy to the very end) said in a letter to her mother, "I'm in good hands. I have a real swashbuckler of an oncologist."

The cancer had advanced throughout her body by this time, leaving little reason to hope for long-term survival, but Blumenschein got her into a clinical trial that combined a variety of drugs with "the red devil," doxorubicin, also known as Adriamycin. The side effects were brutal, but a subclavian catheter installed in her chest during the second round of chemo allowed for the Adria to be administered by continuous infusion, and that made life more manageable.

Suzy's treatment went on for over a year. Her husband, sister, and parents made the long journey with her: shuttle flights, endless driving, waiting rooms, chemo infusion lounges, brief respites beside hotel swimming pools, precious days at home with her children. Dr. Blumenschein became part of this family portrait, responding quickly to changes in Suzy's condition, guiding her through her options, taking the time to make sure her choices were fully informed.

"I won't give up," he kept telling her, "until you tell me to give up."

Suzy died in August of 1980, and some months later, Nancy ran into Dr. Blumenschein at the annual Cattle Baron's Ball, a fundraising gala for the American Cancer Society.

"I'm glad to see you, Dr. B," she said. "I need your advice."

"Fire away."

"I have to cure breast cancer."

He smiled at her and said, "Me too."

I suppose it might have sounded like hyperbole to anyone overhearing this conversation between the bereaved sister and the dedicated oncologist, but both of them were dead serious. Nancy went on to form the foundation named in Suzy's memory. Dr. Blumenschein went on to join with other pioneers in adjuvant therapy, developing treatment protocols in a way that for many women does, in fact, cure breast cancer. Nancy herself is one of his success stories.

Diagnosed with the same type and stage of breast cancer that had killed her sister 3 years earlier, Nancy went immediately to Dr. Blumenschein at M.D. Anderson. Under his watchful eye, she opted for a double mastectomy and adjuvant chemotherapy, and not only did she live to tell about it, she lived to change the world. Over the next 30 years, Susan G. Komen for the Cure rallied millions of volunteers around the globe and raised over $2 billion for breast cancer research, treatment, services and education, changing the perception and experience of breast cancer on a cultural level.

While I was working with Nancy on her memoir, I tried repeatedly to reach Dr. Blumenschein so I could interview him, and it rankled me more than a little that he never got back to me. I assumed that he was a typically arrogant oncologist who didn't have time to bother with the questions of a curious writer, but I found out later that he was struggling to recover from a devastating respiratory collapse following spinal surgery.

"I don't know how much of my book I left on that emergency room floor," he told me recently. "I know I lost something."

The impact of that collapse combined with advancing Parkinson's disease effectively ended his brilliant career.

The loss of Dr. Blumenschein was keenly felt by his patients, who poured out concern and love for him in a pile of letters that are stacked on his dining room table today. I've come to Dallas to work with him on the book you hold in your hand, and it wouldn't be complete without their thoughts:

Dear Dr. Blumenschein,

Recently I had reason to re-read the pathology reports of my breast cancer, from needle aspiration to biopsy to mastectomy. My sister has enrolled in a "Sister Study" of women whose sisters had breast cancer, and she needed some background information. I don't particularly like to revisit that time in my life, but I am an ardent advocate of continuing research.

I am ecstatic and very grateful that I am writing to you almost 22 years later. There is certainly no good statistical reason for me to still be alive. I was fairly young (33), my cancer was ER/PR negative and quite aggressive. You treated me with CAVe, then turned me over to Sam Jampolis for radiation. I refused to follow up with MCCFUD, as I had a small child to raise and a marriage falling apart; I needed my full strength to cope with what time I had left. On my own, I elected to have the other breast removed—more to achieve symmetry than as a prophylactic measure.

And here I am today. Knock wood, there have been no recurrences, and I am in good health. Whatever combination of treatments allowed this to happen, you deserve a huge round of appreciation and approbation. Thank you, Dr. Blumenschein, for working so hard to give me back my life.

Another letter reads:

Dear Dr. Blumenschein,

I was one of your hopeless patients that came to you in 1982 with 4th stage breast cancer. I think of you often and will never forget all you did for me over the years to keep me alive. My husband and I think of you often and your name is mentioned many times as our hero.

My sister, who was also your patient passed away in 2009. We were fortunate to have her alive the 10 years you treated her for liver and bone cancer. She never trusted any other doctor after you retired and lost her interest to fight—she said you were the only doctor that cared.

Another letter reads:

Dear Dr. Blumenschein,

It's with heavy heart that I am writing you today after hearing that you have retired from the Cancer Center. I last saw you in February and you told me that I had made your day after hearing how well I was doing 9 years after my HER-positive cancer diagnosis. I am eternally grateful to you for being there for me when I could so easily have died with that type of cancer, which was positive in nine lymph nodes. During my months of chemo in 1999–2000, I sat by many women who told me their stories of how you had saved their lives and given them hope.

Another letter begins:

Dear Dr. Blumenschein,

It has been 15 years since my breast cancer diagnosis. I feel compelled to write to you at 5-year intervals to thank you for the gift of my life. After consulting with six doctors in Chicago... you were the only doctor who gave me hope. I am here today and value every day I have been given.

As a cancer survivor myself, I'm familiar with the industrial atmosphere of a large cancer treatment center. I understand what this level of care meant to these women—*care* in the truest, most personal sense of that word—but perhaps the most striking characteristic of Dr. Blumenschein's abundantly striking character is a confidently hopeful resilience that was clearly infectious to his patients.

On Nancy's recommendation, Dr. Blumenschein reached out to me about a book of his own. He'd spent some time early in his retirement writing a brief history of the development of adjuvant therapies from his perspective as a young hematologist and later as the head of Breast Services at M.D. Anderson Cancer Center in Houston and Arlington Cancer Center near Dallas.

When I read his short manuscript, I found it very interesting and I hope you will enjoy sitting with this book as greatly as I've enjoyed the privilege of getting to know Dr. Blumenschein.

Joni Rodgers
Dallas, TX
May 2012

This is a brief, slightly autobiographic tale of medical oncologists, surgeons, radiation oncologists, and breast cancer patients in a well-established cancer center in Texas, who pursued the goal of cure for breast cancer, and quite possibly achieved it. The evolution of improved outcomes in the treatment of microscopic metastatic breast cancer is also the story of the development of adjuvant chemotherapy for postoperative breast disease. The adjuvant therapy of breast cancer came about with the realization that this malignancy, when diagnosed in most patients, had spread beyond the confines of the primary.

From time to time, M.D. Anderson Cancer Center (MDA) and Arlington Cancer Center (ACC) patient histories are used to illustrate certain issues. While many have asked to allow their identity and personal information to be disclosed, it is best for all if these are not revealed. So patients' names, exact ages, unimportant social histories, and geographic locations will be fictitious. The natural history of the breast cancer used to illustrate a point, however, will remain as accurate as possible. The author hopes that the information presented in this compilation of chapters and case studies will help empower women with breast cancer to make informed decisions about their various therapeutic options.

The author's use of the third person allows him to appear to be in the thick of the action and helps to chronicle the influence of scientific events, both basic and clinical, and their role in the unexplained luck that so often shapes career decisions. In fact, he considers himself lucky to have been such a close observer of the historic struggle to cure breast cancer.

DISCLAIMER

No part of this book is to be construed or misconstrued as medical advice. Views presented here are those of the author, Dr. George R. Blumenschein, and do not necessarily reflect the views of M.D. Anderson Cancer Center or any other educational, nonprofit, or corporate entity with which the author has been, is now, or will in the future be associated. Persons and events are depicted in accordance with the author's recollection as of this writing with the author's due respect for others whose recollection and/or perception of depicted persons and events may differ from those of the author.

CHAPTER 1

Anatomy of an Oncologist

Dr. George Richard Blumenschein was raised in the modest Chicago suburb of Elmhurst. Following an immensely successful sojourn at York Community High School, he found himself among equals at Yale where he received a BA degree and gained entrance to Cornell University Medical College. During a medical internship at Bellevue Hospital's Cornell Division, he accepted a 2-year appointment to the Epidemic Intelligence Service (EIS) of the United States Public Health Service where he fulfilled the 2 years of military service that were required of physicians trained during the Vietnam era.

It was during those 2 years that he began to develop an overriding interest in cancer. As an EIS officer, he was assigned to Dr. John Moloney's laboratory at the National Cancer Institute (NCI) in Bethesda, MD. This assignment was an amazing stroke of good fortune as the NCI is widely recognized as the "Mother University" of the study of cancer in the United States and, possibly, the world. Here, under Moloney's direction, Blumenschein discovered a new tumor virus, the Moloney Sarcoma Virus. These 2 years were very formative for Blumenschein and, rather than complete the clinical studies necessary to qualify as a practicing physician, he seriously considered pursuing a career in tumor virology.

Common sense prevailed and he spent the next 3 years in Durham, NC at the Duke Hospital completing his training in internal medicine, immunology, and hematology (oncology did not exist as a subspecialty in medicine until 1973). In 1969, an opportunity arose at Northwestern University Medical School to develop a subsection of medical oncology, and Blumenschein moved his growing family to Chicago. Blumenschein maintained a busy schedule as Northwestern's first medical oncologist. He continued to explore the transfer of immunity to Moloney Sarcoma, developed an oncology elective for medical students (of the six students who took the elective, all six later became medical oncologists), and became a principal consultant for oncology referral to the practicing medical community. To assist in patient referrals, he also joined

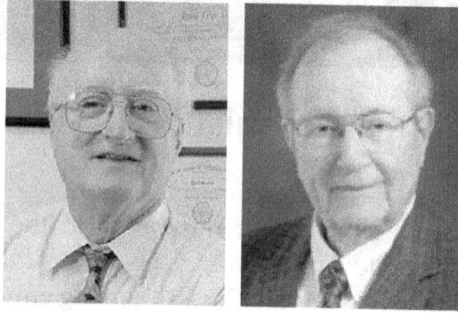

Figure 1.1 The two Emils who inspired and mentored Blumenschein. Dr. Emil J Freireich on the right (Photograph courtesy of Barry Smith, Department of Medical Graphics & Photography, The University of Texas MD Anderson Cancer Center) and Dr. Emil Frei, III on the left (Photograph courtesy Steve Gilbert, Harvard Medical School).

Southwest Oncology Group (SWOG), a multi-institutional clinical trials group that gave him access to investigational treatment protocols and clinical trials of new drugs.

As his interest in oncology became more focused, his interest was drawn to the activities of two giants in the field, Drs. Emil J Freireich and Emil Frei III (Figure 1.1), whose pursuits covered a wide spectrum of subject matter associated with oncology, ranging from basic science, to supportive care, statistics, pharmacology, immunology, and chemotherapy. Drs. Freireich and Frei had been recruited from the NCI to M. D. Anderson (MDA) where they had formed the country's first Department of Developmental Therapeutics. They worked well together and were responsible for establishing the clinical principles that underlie contemporary oncologic practice. They shared the same first name by chance and, from time to time, this caused considerable confusion. In an amusing instance, Dr. Freireich was being presented to the body of the American Association for Cancer Research as its newly elected president. Following completion of his presidential lecture, he was presented with, among other things, a handsomely engraved bronze plaque commemorating the occasion. On reading the inscription, Freireich began to chuckle and showed it to the audience. The plaque was inscribed to Emil J Freireich, III.

While Blumenschein's interest in clinical medical oncology and his reputation waxed at Northwestern, his concern about his laboratory projects and the viral-induced sarcoma waned. Despite his success, Blumenschein felt that his training in oncology was deficient and that he needed to move on to obtain in-depth exposure to individuals, such as Drs. Freireich and Frei. On the other hand, Blumenschein felt he needed to consider his beautiful and accomplished wife Sarah, whose career in pediatric cardiology was moving along nicely, even though she was in her fourth pregnancy. They each had family roots in the Chicago area, as well.

1.1 NEXT STOP—MDA

MDA is a unique care and research facility focusing on cancer. It is located in a large medical center complex together with Baylor University Medical School, The University of Texas Health Science Center, and the Texas Heart Institute. Its genesis dates to the passage of a bill by the state legislature in 1927 to develop a facility to care for people with cancer, pellagra, and insanity. The bill was not funded due to the Great Depression and World War II, but in 1947, the Ways and Means Committee funded the project and established the cancer hospital in six Army surplus Quonset huts at the upper end of Houston's Herman Park.

The search committee to recommend a head for MDA was chaired by Texas governor Allan Shivers. He decreed that the head of the cancer facility should be a cancer authority, preferably a Texan, and a surgeon. He felt this person should report to the governor through the university system rather than the health department or a free-standing department. By placing MDA in the University of Texas system, academic titles could be included in the recruitment package for physicians. This improved the quality of the physician researchers that were recruited.

In 1946, the search committee chose Dr. R. Lee Clark to be the first full-time director and surgeon-in-chief of MDA. Dr. Clark was born and raised in north central Texas. His maternal grandmother's second husband was Robert E. Lee's younger brother. Her first husband had been killed by Comanches while he was plowing his field. After completing medical school in Virginia and 5 years of surgical residency, Dr. Clark took a fellowship in surgical oncology at the Mayo Clinic in Rochester, MN. Thus, he was eminently qualified to head MDA. Dr. Clark entered the army medical corps and spent World War II in the European theater. Following the war, and a year as Head of the American Hospital in Paris, he established a successful surgical practice in Jackson, MS. This is

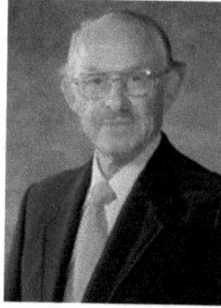

Figure 1.2 R. Lee Clark, M.D. who served from 1946 to 1968 as Director and from 1968 to 1978 as President of MDA. (Photograph courtesy of the Department of Medical Graphics & Photography, The University of Texas MD Anderson Cancer Center).

where Governor Shivers discovered Dr. Clark and identified him as the perfect candidate for the position (Figure 1.2).

During his initial negotiations with the Texas governor, Dr. Clark established for the MDA its form, rules of governance, faculty requirements, structure, and goals. It was to be the equivalent of a free-standing health science unit in the University of Texas, whose basic science and clinical departments and faculty carried out research, patient care, and education on cancer. From the beginning, MDA had a Spartan vertical administrative operating structure. Most decisions were discussed and made by an administrative council which met at least weekly to deal with issues. The council consisted of the President of MDA, Dr. R. Lee Clark, the Director of the Institution, and three Associate Directors, one each for Research, Clinical Affairs, and Education.

Dr. Clark made an interesting arrangement for his salary. He asked for 1000 dollars more per year than the highest salary paid to any state employee. The governor (the state's highest paid employee) annually received $35,000. Dr. Clark signed on for a starting salary of $36,000. This was a bargain for the state of Texas as Dr. Clark had earned $150,000 over 2 years prior to closing his surgical practice in Jackson.

In 1950, the Monroe Dunaway Anderson Foundation, established by a successful cotton broker in Houston, donated 4 million dollars to the cancer facility. This was used to replace the 6 army surplus Quonset huts that initially housed the facility with a 5-story 220-bed hospital and outpatient cancer treatment facility covered by pink marble from a quarry seen by Dr. Clark when he was backpacking through Georgia as a medical school student. The Anderson family's generosity was recognized by the naming of the cancer center and also enabled MDA, as a state-owned and operated facility, to subsidize the care of Texas citizens according to need.

The institution was blessed with two medicine departments, the first dating to the founding of MDA. However, none of the faculty in this original internal medicine department possessed a background in clinical research related to cancer. Chemotherapy was limited and strategies to amplify drug efficacy were in their infancy. By 1965, the picture was beginning to change, principally due to the investment of time and money by the NCI and the tireless efforts of Drs. Freireich and Frei and other brilliant physician scientists. Dr. Clark took notice of the growing importance of chemotherapy for cancer treatment and offered Freireich and Frei the opportunity to come to MDA to develop a department of medicine that emphasized clinical research in cancer treatment. This second department of medicine was appropriately named Developmental Therapeutics.

In 1972, the Associate Director for Education at MDA resigned. Blumenschein was pleased but puzzled when he received a call from Dr. Clark to visit Houston to look at the position. He had never met Dr. Clark and had no prior association with MDA. Despite his admiration for Dr. Freireich, he never had the opportunity to meet him. This was a critical moment for Blumenschein's career. Ever since he had set his cap for oncology, he had wanted to have some meaningful association with Freireich and MDA. Unfortunately, the Associate Director for Education position appeared to be somewhat peripheral to MDA's patient care and research mission. He eventually realized that the title of Associate Director and his seat on the governing council would give him immediate peer status in MDA as he pursued a medical oncology career. So he accepted the position with the stipulation that he be given control of the entire education and training budget and receive an appointment as Assistant Professor, Medical Breast Service, in both departments of medicine.

The conditions accepted, Blumenschein began his sojourn at MDA in February 1973, one month after Sarah gave birth to their fourth child. He was surprised to hear no objection to these conditions from Dr. Freireich, who had a reputation for being careful to not compromise the quality of his faculty by recruiting unproven and untested staff. Fortunately, Blumenschein found Freireich to be very accessible and subsequently sought his counsel whenever possible.

1.2 EARLY EXPERIENCE WITH 5-FLUOROURACIL, ADRIAMYCIN, AND CYCLOPHOSPHAMIDE

The Medical Breast Service in 1973 was a shambles in need of major updating in the modern management of all stages of the disease. There were many patients with untreated advanced disease referred each year from Texas and neighboring states. Each medicine department had its own training program, but the distribution of breast cancer patients was very uneven, favoring the original department, due to well-established habits of referral. Blumenschein addressed this problem by combining the two programs when the issue was breast cancer. He insisted on using a common protocol and sharing a common outpatient space. The major benefit from combining the two breast cancer programs was a significant increase in the amount of clinical data available to each trainee. As part of their training, each fellow was expected to write an original paper utilizing data generated at MDA. This resulted in the annual publication of a large number of abstracts and papers on the subject of breast cancer.

In the summer of 1968, doxorubicin (better known by its trade name Adriamycin) was first approved for clinical use and in 1972–73 became available for treatment of advanced breast cancer (Figure 1.3). While at Northwestern, Blumenschein had used it as a

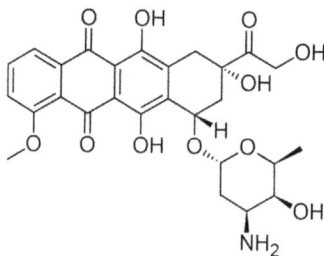

Figure 1.3 Chemical structure of Adriamycin (doxorubicin), technically classified as an anthracycline antibiotic. Adriamycin is formed in nature by Streptomyces peucetius and was initially isolated from a sample of soil found at Castel del Monte, a 13th century castle located near the Adriatic Sea, for which the compound is named. Adriamycin inhibits the proliferation of cancer and other rapidly growing cells (e.g. bone marrow and hair follicles) by fitting itself between base pairs of adjacent strands of DNA, a mechanism termed intercalation.

single agent for the treatment of breast cancer resistant to standard therapy that included cyclophosphamide, methotrexate, 5-fluorouracil, vincristine, and prednisone (abbreviated to CMFVP-resistant disease) and had found it to have significant activity. He suspected it would show even greater effectiveness in combination with other drugs and sought Dr. Freireich's advice as to how to proceed. Freireich suggested that Dr. Geoffrey Gottlieb become involved, and shortly thereafter, Gottlieb put together a protocol consisting of 5-fluorouracil (5FU), Adriamycin, and cyclophosphamide (FAC).

Initially, FAC was administered intravenously in a 28-day schedule. 5FU was given on days 1 and 8; Adriamycin and cyclophosphamide were given on day 1. The dose of each drug was, respectively, 5FU 400 mg/m^2, Adriamycin 40 mg/m^2, and cyclophosphamide 400 mg/m^2. Each patient was monitored for infection, absolute granulocyte count, platelet count, and the degree of nausea, vomiting and hair loss. The electrocardiogram (EKG) was evaluated prior to each Adriamycin dose because there is cumulative myocardial damage associated with the use of this drug. Principally because of concern about cardiac muscle damage, the total dose of Adriamycin was limited to 450 mg/m^2.

Beginning in April 1973, Blumenschein enforced the assignment of stage IV breast cancer patients who were candidates for chemotherapy to the FAC protocol. The use of FAC as adjuvant therapy was initiated that same month. Patient accrual was rapid, tumor response better than expected, and toxicity was manageable. The only nonanthracycline drug combination available for historical response comparison was cyclophosphamide, methotrexate, and 5FU (CMF), a drug combination derived from CMFVP which had activity beyond that of single-agent therapy for breast cancer. An assessment of the first 30 patients with metastatic breast disease who were treated with FAC showed that they responded approximately 75% of the time and had a 20% complete remission rate, compared to the 50% partial remission rate and 5% complete remission rate that had previously been obtained with CMF. More important was the complete lack of tumor growth during the first 2 months of FAC therapy. This had not been the case with CMF-treated patients with metastatic disease, who experienced a 15% chance of cancer progression during that time.

The price paid for this increase in metastatic disease regression from FAC was notable, but manageable. Nausea and vomiting followed Adriamycin administration and the platelet count would reach its nadir by day 10. However, of greatest concern, the absolute granulocyte count would crater around day 13, putting the patient at risk for developing an overwhelming systemic infection. Countermeasures were created to deal with all of these events so that they did not interfere with the prescribed dose and dose rate, or schedule of chemotherapy administration. However, there was nothing Blumenschein or the fellows on the medical breast service could offer to prevent complete hair loss, usually by day 17, and, of a more serious nature at that time, the cumulative damage to the heart muscle with each course of FAC that was later shown to be the result of the high peak plasma concentration of Adriamycin that occurred when this drug was administered by rapid, rather than prolonged, intravenous infusion.

The parameter of response that encouraged these physicians to push on was the improvement in complete remission. Only by achieving complete disappearance of all measurable and microscopic metastatic disease could these medical oncologists dream of achieving *cure*. If a patient had been diagnosed with stage IV breast cancer, defined as metastatic disease, and was treated only with the chemotherapy that was standard in 1973, cure was not even remotely feasible. Microscopic metastases could be present anywhere in the body and could not be clinically detected until they had grown to contain at least 1 billion cells. Thus, the spread of cancer from the primary to other types of tissue could result in an occult metastasis containing from two cells, to a barely detectable mass containing 1 billion cells that might measure 1 cm in diameter. In each of these instances, the patient would be considered to have metastatic disease which, if left untreated, would, through cell division, increase the number of cancer cells and eventually kill the patient. Furthermore, as the number of cells grew, they would change qualitatively and evolve clones that were resistant to the drugs in use at that time.

If metastatic cancer was sensitive to a drug combination and regressed from measurable to unmeasurable as a result of treatment, one had a complete remission, not a cure. Only by the passage of a to-be-determined period of time would one begin to entertain thoughts of cure. In 1974, as it would be today, it was impossible to discern if a patient in complete remission contained either 0 or just under 1 billion remaining cancer cells.

One would assume that the most effective drug combination for achieving complete remission when treating measurable metastases also would be chosen as the chemotherapy combination to use as adjuvant therapy in the post-mastectomy setting, where metastatic disease is not measurable. For some reasons, the majority of adjuvant treatment programs had avoided the most active drug against breast cancer: Adriamycin. The reasons given for ignoring its use usually were (1) the drug is too toxic for adjuvant use; (2) nothing of its activity will remain to help the patient after the disease has recurred on Adriamycin; (3) we've not been trained in its use; (4) a patient with no measurable metastatic disease should not have to experience the same horrific side effects as the one with lethal metastatic cancer; (5) it may be necessary to hire additional personnel to administer the drug and care for the immediate side effects; and (6) there is no randomized clinically similar group receiving CMF concurrently, to use as a control population. Fortunately, the Medical Breast Service and Developmental Therapeutics Department had an opportunity to analyze the results of the first 30 patients with metastatic breast cancer who were treated with FAC and were impressed with the results cited above. Clearly, there was but one choice for a chemotherapy program to offer MDA patients for the adjuvant treatment of breast cancer.

1.3 MONDAY NIGHT CONFRONTATION

In July 1973, Dr. Aman Buzdar completed his fellowship in medical oncology and joined Blumenschein as a clinician and faculty member on the medical breast service. Later that summer, Dr. Gabriel Hortobagyi did the same. There was a great deal of interest and enthusiasm about breast cancer at that time because of the increasing evidence of the sensitivity of this highly prevalent solid tumor to chemotherapy combinations. The incidence of the disease was increasing annually and a large amount of data was being collected. The Medical Breast Service at MDA grew rapidly as its reputation for aggressive treatment of a serious disease became more widely known. However, apparently not everyone at MDA was impressed with the performance of this young newcomer from Northwestern. In a year's time, he had, while carrying out his responsibilities in education, obtained the top grant in the country for cancer education, usurped the medical breast program, blurred the division between the two medicine departments with respect to breast cancer, and encroached on radiation therapy and surgical territory with regard to breast cancer management.

This rapid success was bound to "ruffle some feathers" but the major focus of articulated concern swirled around the use of Adriamycin. So on a Monday afternoon, the heads of the departments of surgery, medicine, radiation therapy, radiology, and gynecology, and the chief of the medical breast service went to Dr. Clark's office and unloaded their complaints about Blumenschein and Adriamycin. After hearing the chorus of complaints, Dr. Clark summoned Blumenschein from the Breast Clinic to his office to hear the litany of concerns. The majority of issues that the senior staff raised had to do with Adriamycin toxicity that could be managed. However, they were not accustomed to the sight of ill patients who had experienced complete hair loss and they feared the risks being taken with cardiac injury. Clark asked Blumenschein to respond. Fortunately, he could point out that the first 30 patients with metastatic breast cancer treated with FAC had benefited with an unprecedented 20% complete remission rate and enjoyed an overall response rate of 75%. When Blumenschein came to his office the following morning, he found a memo from Dr. Clark indicating that, as of that day, he was to assume the position of Chief of the Medical Breast Service.

Overnight, Blumenschein had become an instant authority on breast cancer. But he had much to learn.

Case Study

Janet

Highly Sensitive, Measurable Metastatic Breast Cancer

The extent of Dr. Blumenschein's practice was very large and included over 2000 patients. Consequently, the spectrum of tumor activity in these patients was diverse and heterogeneous. At the most favorable end of the spectrum were patients with well-differentiated, slow growing, and drug-sensitive cancer clones in whom a complete remission could be obtained with chemotherapy alone.

Janet, a 56-year-old administrative assistant, had been diagnosed with advanced primary breast cancer in her left breast. The cancer had metastasized to her lungs, liver, bone, and axillary and supraclavicular lymph nodes. Her primary physician was alarmed and started her on a course of FAC. She was ready for her second course of FAC when she was seen by Blumenschein. His physical examination indicated that she had already begun to respond to FAC. Her lungs were clear, her lymph nodes had regressed, and the mass in her left breast had vanished. Her liver had decreased in size and her liver function tests also had begun to improve. Staging studies confirmed these findings.

Therefore, Blumenschein continued the FAC regimen for a total of nine courses during which her bone lesions showed blastic healing. Subsequently, he elected to follow her at 3-month intervals for the next 5 years. At that point, follow-up visits were scheduled every 6 months. After 10 years, he saw her annually. Blumenschein considers Janet to have been cured, but because blastic healing of bone lesions occurs in the absence of radiologic change she is technically classified as being in stable partial remission rather than in complete remission.

Case Study

Susan

The Importance of Axillary Node Involvement

The number of ipsilateral axillary nodes involved with breast cancer has become an increasingly important consideration in planning an attack on a patient's primary disease. However, the use of the sentinel node technique[1] for purposes of staging the extent of the primary breast disease is sometimes problematic. A clinical example will explain the dilemma that can be caused by a misreading of the axillary node situation. If N_0 (absence of identified lymph nodes with cancer) is really N_1 (cancer metastases found in one or more axillary lymph nodes), inappropriate therapy will be chosen.

Susan Cole, a widow at age 38, owned and operated a chain of pharmacies in the Chicago suburbs. There was no prior history of cancer in her family. She was healthy and fit and enjoyed an active social life. Her current love interest was a young surgeon who had been recently divorced. After a fun evening at the Art Institute of Chicago, he escorted her home. In the ensuing course of events, he palpated a mass in the upper outer quadrant of her left breast and was forced to assume the role of physician. She could tell he was concerned, and the evening ended after he explained what she must do immediately.

The following morning she called her gynecologist and asked his advice. He referred her to Dr. Gerald Powell, a general surgeon in practice at Northwestern Memorial Hospital and he ordered a mammogram. She had a lesion in the described location and underwent an ultrasound-guided core biopsy. There was no doubt about the diagnosis, and she and Dr. Powell had a lengthy discussion as to how to proceed. He favored a standard mastectomy, principally to assure adequate staging. But Susan, being single and not wanting to lose her breast, convinced the surgeon to remove the lump and any nearby suspicious nodes followed by whole breast irradiation.

The surgery was uneventful. The cancer measured 2.3 cm in diameter. There was perilymphatic invasion in the area of the cancer. One of five left axillary (sentinel) lymph nodes was histologically positive for metastatic spread. The cancer was estrogen and progesterone receptor negative (ER−, PR−). At this point, Susan mentioned that, "by the way", she would like a referral to Dr. Blumenschein in Arlington, TX.

---

[1]The sentinel note technique is one in which patients are injected in the area of the tumor with a saline solution of technetium-labeled colloid 2−16 h before surgery and with isosulfan blue dye at the time of surgery. Sentinel lymph nodes, identified by their presence of radioactivity and blue staining, are removed for microscopic evaluation of metastatic tumor.

Blumenschein did not like the tumor's perilymphatic invasion and convinced Susan that Dr. Powell was correct. He felt that the limited nodal evaluation may have incorrectly downstaged Susan to stage II with *less* than three positive nodes with an expected 80% chance of cure. This would have permitted her to qualify for less therapy than she actually needed if she had been classified as stage II with *more* than three positive nodes. In that case, there would be concern that starting with radiation therapy would delay the time to chemotherapy by about 10–12 weeks and give any microscopic foci of metastases outside the radiation field time to grow and exceed a size that chemotherapy could eliminate, i.e., <1 million cells. Unfortunately, this level of sophistication was not common when therapeutic planning for Susan took place 23 years ago.

For some reasons, Susan decided to remain in Arlington for the mastectomy and lymph node evaluation that Blumenschein recommended. Dr. Bohn Allen was very accommodating, saw Susan immediately, and made arrangements for surgery to be done on the following day. The results were not what her referring physician had expected. Dr. Allen found 17 additional lymph nodes containing cancer. So Susan's prognosis changed dramatically to less than a 20% chance of 5-year survival. The recommended treatment changed to induction with 6 courses of FAC (abbreviated as FAC × 6) to be followed by a combination of methotrexate, cisplatin, Cytoxan (trade name for cyclophosphamide), and 5FU with leucovorin for methotrexate rescue (MCCFUD) × 3. Chest wall and peripheral lymphatic irradiation was begun 4 weeks after MCCFUD.

For the 5 years following January 1988, Susan was seen by Blumenschein every 3 months. Visits to Texas then gradually diminished to every 4 months, then every 6 months. January 1995 could be considered a close call when symptoms of a headache led to the discovery of a dural mass. Fortunately, this proved to be a meningioma that was successfully resected 2 months later. Today, Susan is continuing to enjoy life in Chicago and is sharing it with the surgeon who had been her date on that Art Institute evening.

Blumenschein considers that Susan has been cured and that FAC was the modality that successfully eradicated her microscopic metastatic disease. Although regional radiation therapy may have contributed somewhat to her cure, it is not clear in retrospect that MCCFUD was necessary.

CHAPTER 2

Milestones Along the Road to the Cure

If the goal of every cancer patient today is cure, does oncology have, in its medical bag of tricks, sufficient understanding of the biology of a human cell gone astray, the medications to control such behavior, and the wisdom and courage to attain this goal? The answer for breast cancer is yes. Following is a review of the evolution of the significant, and not so significant, efforts and milestones that went into achieving the goal of curing breast cancer. These have occurred over the past 40 years and have involved the participation and sacrifice of untold numbers of patients. The knowledge gained has now given the patient's physician, and the patient, the power to correctly direct therapeutic decisions.

The search for an effective chemotherapy regimen began when empirical evidence led to the obvious conclusion that eradication of the disease might best be achieved when it was in microscopic quantities. So it was evident this therapy needed to be given as an adjunctive to surgery and/or radiation that could be directed toward the visible sites of tumor involvement (Figure 2.1). The discovery and development of active individual chemotherapeutic drugs and study of anticancer drug combinations were central in this effort. Also essential to this progress were advances in the fundamental understanding of cancer cell biology and the elucidation of prognostic indicators to guide therapeutic strategy.

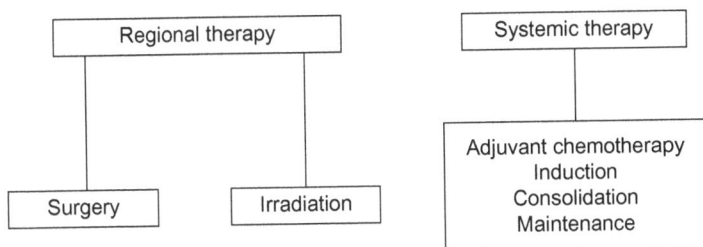

```
┌─────────────────────────┐        ┌─────────────────────────┐
│    Regional therapy     │        │    Systemic therapy     │
└─────────────────────────┘        └─────────────────────────┘
       │          │                            │
   ┌───────┐  ┌───────────┐        ┌─────────────────────────┐
   │Surgery│  │Irradiation│        │ Adjuvant chemotherapy   │
   └───────┘  └───────────┘        │      Induction          │
                                   │     Consolidation       │
                                   │      Maintenance        │
                                   └─────────────────────────┘
```

Figure 2.1 Contemporary strategy for treating patients with breast cancer combines the regional approaches of surgery and radiation therapy, directed toward towards tumor areas that can be visualized, with systemic administration of adjuvant chemotherapy that is most effective against microscopic foci of metastatic disease. In some cases, adjuvant induction therapy is followed by additional consolidation and/or maintenance chemotherapy.

2.1 THE IMPORTANCE OF PATIENT EDUCATION

Another essential aspect of curing patients with breast cancer is their education, which should begin with their first visit to their participating physician, usually a medical oncologist. It is important for that physician to get to know the patient and to ascertain her basic understanding of cell biology and cancer. Every breast cancer patient should have a healthy grounding in the biology that got her there, so she can better understand her options and the *why*s of what we prescribe. A patient engaged in her care will be more compliant and usually will have a more successful outcome. The following is a brief summary of information that patients should have.

Breast cancer is essentially a disease of organized cell growth and function gone awry. Cancer cells no longer follow the direction of their neighbors. Once they transform, they have a tendency to revert to even more erratic behavior. It is believed by most pathologists that ductal breast cancer begins with well-behaved intraductal cells, cells lining the milk ducts, which for some reason are injured to the degree that they no longer recognize the constraint placed on all mature, differentiated cells to not divide. When a cell, or group of cells, begins dividing without normal constraints, both their rate of division and rate of mutation increase. A transformed cell has certain recognizable characteristics, or "hallmarks" which give it a competitive advantage over the neighboring cells in its microenvironment. Such cells are able to not only induce growth of their blood supply, termed angiogenesis, and activate invasion but also can reprogram energy metabolism to sustain proliferative signaling and evade growth suppressors, so as to resist cell death and thereby achieve replicative immortality.[1]

In addition, the genomic instability of cancer cells leads to genetic diversity and the emergence of cell clones that are resistant to chemotherapy. An early cancer also will eventually undergo mutations that allow it to divide relentlessly and to no longer stop at the boundaries of adjacent cells. Invasion into the space of other cells occurs. After invasion is established, spread to other tissues is possible. Clumps of cancer cells dislodge and float downstream through veins, cross from the right to the left side of the heart, to alight in other organs and proceed with more division in these new locations. Eventually, one or

---

[1]Hanahan D, Weinberg RA. Hallmarks of cancer: the next generation. Cell 2011;144:646–74.

more groups will increase to a number that exceeds 1 billion cells so that they become visible. These are known as metastases and represent at least 27 generations of divisions of an initial cancer cell. Metastases indicate a poor prognosis. In the past, when metastases were discovered in a patient, she was classified as stage IV and had little hope for long-term survival. But this is no longer true.

Within every stage of advanced breast cancer there are substages that reflect the number of metastatic cells that may be present, either more than 1 billion cells in the early macro range or less than 1 billion cells in the micro range. Examples of substages of advanced breast cancer are better known as stage II with >10 positive nodes, stage III, stage IV with no evidence of disease (NED), surgical complete remission, or radiation therapy-induced complete remission, stage IV chemotherapy-induced complete remission, and inflammatory breast cancer (IBC). Each of these substages has a high probability of developing metastases after the usual initial therapy. An understanding of the natural history of several subsets of patients with these advanced substages of breast cancer played an important role in studying the impact of various adjuvant therapies on their outcomes.

Equally important was the realization that the accelerated rate at which cancer cells divide is what makes them susceptible to chemotherapeutic agents that, in general, block the molecular machinery that is involved in their proliferation. Unfortunately, this action also results in toxicity because rapidly proliferating normal cells, such as those in the bone marrow, are also vulnerable. The advantages of combination chemotherapy are that it counteracts the ability of cancer cells to mutate and become chemotherapy resistant and it also achieves therapeutic efficacy by using less toxic doses of each agent in the combination than would be required with single-agent therapy. These fundamental concepts provided a sound therapeutic rationale for the development adjuvant chemotherapy.

Patients come to an oncologist's office because they believe that medicine has the tools, the strategies, and the drugs to eliminate every last cancer cell. The question being asked by some oncologists was, "If it is possible to cure some of these stage IV and advanced stage II and III breast cancers, why are we not trying these strategies and drugs on all such patients?" For if cure is not our goal, then surely we shall fail in every attempt. Therefore, the patient with advanced breast cancer has a particular need to be educated about her options. The initial visit should therefore be lengthy and largely structured to inform the patient about where oncology has come from and how good outcomes are accomplished. After this introduction, the oncologist should switch to the specifics of the particular patient and outline an approach to possibly solve her dilemma. If we fail, what difference would it have made from not trying at all?

2.2 PIONEERS OF ADJUVANT THERAPY

The development of a program to cure breast cancer paralleled the evolution of the development of adjuvant chemotherapy to improve outcomes in breast cancer patients postmastectomy. Three men stand out as leaders in this effort: Dr. Bernard Fisher, Professor of Surgery, University of Pittsburgh, Dr. Gianni Bonadonna, Professor of Medicine, University of Milan, and Dr. Aman Buzdar, Professor of Medicine, University of Texas-MDA. Each is associated with a regimen and strategy that moved the field forward in this endeavor: Dr. Fisher, melphalan (L-PAM), 5-FU; Dr. Bonadonna, CMF; Dr. Buzdar, FAC, with special emphasis directed toward Adriamycin. Similar chemotherapeutic agents, but not necessarily similar strategies, were used by these investigators in the attempt to eradicate every last cancer cell.

In 1957, Dr. Fisher initiated the national interest in the use of chemotherapy to enhance patient response to mastectomy by establishing the National Surgical Adjuvant Breast Program (NSABP) to ensure, as best he could, accuracy and quantity in the data collection. With a fluctuating roster of clinical investigators and a smoothly functioning central office, Dr. Fisher forged ahead, conducting clinical trials on a multitude of questions concerning adjuvant therapy. One of the overriding issues in designing these clinical investigations was that they were to be properly controlled by randomly assigning patients to each treatment arm that was being compared.

2.3 EARLY STUDIES

There was some curiosity about the NSABP's choice of L-PAM as its initial chemotherapeutic drug for study. L-PAM was selected for the "kick-off" NSABP trial because it could be given with little interference with a patient's normal routine; it was taken by mouth and caused little nausea and no hair loss. Unfortunately, its activity against measurable metastatic breast cancer was marginal. Early on, the clinical trials showed that combining surgery, usually a Halsted radical mastectomy, with either L-PAM or thiotepa resulted in limited benefit to the patient. Postmenopausal women with metastatic disease seemed to do best. However, Dr. Bernard Fisher in 1968 reported a statistically significant but modest increase in 5-year survival of *premenopausal* stage II patients with >3 positive axillary lymph nodes treated with surgery and single-agent L-PAM.

In 1969, Dr. Richard Cooper from Buffalo reported at a meeting of the American Society of Clinical Oncology (ASCO) that adjuvant therapy with CMFVP resulted in a 68% rate of remission in patients with metastatic breast cancer. Cooper's report generated a great deal of excitement in the fledgling field of medical oncology by, in essence, announcing that breast cancer was a malignancy with increased sensitivity to therapy when *multiple* agents were given together. This was a major paradigm shift!

During his prolific career, Dr. Bonadonna conducted a myriad of clinical trials in Milan that established the essential principles to be followed in the design and conduct of cancer chemotherapy trials. In 1972, he simplified CMFVP to just include CMF. This three-drug regimen could be given to outpatients with a 4-week schedule and had very manageable toxicity. Outcomes with CMF were very reproducible and reliable. Fifty percent of patients with metastatic breast cancer achieved a partial remission, 5% had a complete remission, and only 15% progressed during the first 3 months of treatment.

The development of the FAC protocol at MDA represented a further therapeutic advance and the Medical Breast Service and Developmental Therapeutics Department rapidly determined the superior activity of this regimen in treating patients with metastatic breast cancer. There also was no hesitation at MDA in using this same regimen to treat microscopic breast disease. Dr. Buzdar took charge of this project and entered his first patient on the FAC adjuvant study in January 1974. He subsequently guided its modification, defended its efficacy and reliability, and reported its outcomes on an almost annual basis. With each assessment of relapse-free survival, overall survival, and risk of developing metastases, there was a gain for all of the subsets: node-negative; node-positive; tumor sizes (T) 1,2,3; number of nodes (N) with metastases $N_1 = 1 - 3$, $N_2 = 4 - 10$, $N_3 > 10$; and in both pre- and postmenopausal women. Any comparisons that were done against CMF showed a 12–15% reduction in recurrence rate and death rates when FAC was the induction adjuvant program.

Joan M. Bull at the NCI and Richard V. Smalley at Temple in Philadelphia confirmed these results by each independently conducting clinical trials to compare the efficacy of CMF with that of FAC in patients with metastatic breast cancer. Patients were randomized in each trial to receive one combination or the other and each trial proclaimed FAC the winner. However, there had to be a difference in the conduct of the trials because the response rate to FAC in the Smalley study turned out to be the same as the response to CMF in the Bull study (Figure 2.2). This is one of the best examples to argue for within-trial randomization of patients to treatment when comparing different drug regimens. But Buzdar could not bring himself to recommend randomization to patients who had come to MDA for the "best" treatment. So he used statistically less rigorous *historical* controls to give the Medical Breast Service some assurance that they were not running off the track and drawing erroneous conclusions. This use of historical controls instead of randomization for patient selection in MDA's Adriamycin breast adjuvant studies caused Dr. Buzdar and his

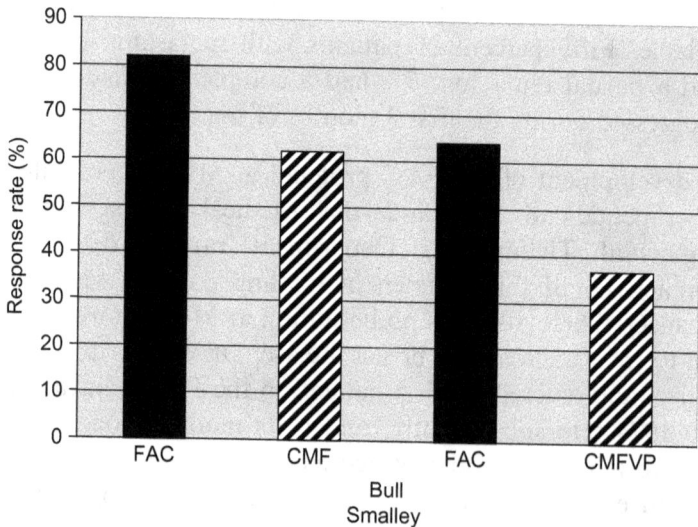

Figure 2.2 Response rates to FAC and CMF combination chemotherapy regimens reported by Bull and Smalley. The Smalley group added vincristine (V) and prednisone (P) to their CMF regimen. (Data from Bull JM, et al. Cancer 1978;41:1649-57 and Smalley RV, et al. Cancer 1977;40:625–32.)

close associates, Drs. Hortobagyi and Blumenschein, no end of grief. The following exchange is an example of this sort of difficulty.

When substituting for Dr. Buzdar at an international meeting on the subject of the adjuvant treatment of operable breast cancer, Dr. Blumenschein was taken to task for MDA's clinical trials utilizing Adriamycin. The meeting was being held in London and had a large European audience. Blumenschein thought he was going to present a 10-year update that Dr. Buzdar had recently completed on his 1973, 222-patient FAC trial. The control population consisted of 186 patients treated at MDA who were node-positive and were selected retrospectively from those treated prior to 1973. They received only mastectomy and radiation therapy and were followed prospectively. Sometime prior to an 8-year update, Dr. Buzdar extended the control population to make it more comparable in numbers to the FAC-treated patients. This had no impact on the prognostic comparability of the two groups. Dr. Buzdar's reports were always anticipated with interest because his results with the aggressive FAC adjuvant regimen were years ahead of the pack. However, what many considered to be the premature utilization of a toxic drug in an adjuvant trial, the absence of concurrently treated randomized controls, and the increase in the number of historic controls midstream, so to speak, was a clinical trial designer's "perfect storm."

Dr. Steven Carter was a highly respected leader in the design and management of cancer clinical trials. His presentation immediately preceded Blumenschein's. Each presentation was to be given over 15 min, reserving 5 min for questions and discussion. Dr. Carter warmed to his topic: "The Design and Conduct of a Clinical Drug Trial." The further along he got, the more he focused on the study Blumenschein was about to present as an example of how not to do one. He overran his total allotted time of 20 min, so the discussion period was omitted and Blumenschein had no time for rebuttal.

As Blumenschein strode from the rear of the auditorium to the podium, the audience was hushed. A vigorous response would be required. Not just vigorous, he realized; it would have to be clever. As he adjusted the microphone and grasped the podium, a response with proper vigor and humor materialized. "Before I begin the presentation," he said, "I find it necessary to respond to Dr. Carter's discussion of Dr. Buzdar's updated review of FAC adjuvant therapy of stage

II–III node-positive breast cancer, initiated in 1973. Dr. Carter is a designer and implementer of clinical trials, a clinical investigator. Dr. Buzdar and I are physicians. Every time I am asked to comment on Dr. Carter's criticism of our work, I think of the response of Earl Butts (Nixon's Secretary of Agriculture) to the question of what he thought about the Pope's position on birth control. His politically insensitive answer cost him his job: "*Ifa youa don'ta playa the gamea, youa don'ta makea the rulesa.*" There was silence, then laughter, followed by applause. Dr. Carter left to catch a plane, and Dr. Blumenschein launched into his presentation.

Dr. Buzdar's outcome reports for the adjuvant chemotherapy with Adriamycin combinations of all of the multiple stages of postoperative breast cancer were unquestionably the best in the country and probably the world. In his initial 1976 abstract describing FAC adjuvant therapy, he reported that both pre- and postmenopausal patients with positive nodes had an increased relapse-free survival. His follow-up analysis in 1980 was again measured against historic controls. So despite its superiority, it was not recognized by the panel that prepared the First Consensus Report because it lacked randomized controls. Seeing this omission from the panel's conclusions and recommendations, one of the panel members asked to present a minority position. She was an attractive lady with a head full of red curls and was on the panel as a consumer representative. She made the following remark in objecting to the lack of recognition of FAC by the panel:

> Three years ago, when I was 28, I was diagnosed with a stage III breast cancer. The tumor was large and 8 axillary nodes were involved with cancer. I am here today because my oncologist insisted I receive FAC adjuvant therapy.

2.4 M.D. ANDERSON: A PIONEER IN RADIATION THERAPY

Dr. R. Lee Clark spent the final year of his military service as chief medical officer at the American Hospital in Paris. There he befriended a young Frenchman, Dr. Gilbert Fletcher, who was on his way toward establishing a significant reputation in the use of irradiation for treating cancer patients. So when Dr. Clark came to MDA, he recruited Fletcher to develop the radiation therapy program and a training fellowship in radiation oncology. Subsequently, MDA was the first hospital in the United States to acquire a cobalt unit, and linear accelerators of much higher energy were soon to follow. Much of the evidence to support the significant role that MDA currently plays in treating patients with breast cancer was developed by Fletcher and the staff that he trained at MDA.

When Dr. Clark arrived at MDA, he was also aware of the growing importance of chemotherapy for treating patients with cancer. So after recruiting Drs. Freireich and Frei and establishing the Developmental Therapeutics Department, MDA was well positioned to investigate the use of chemotherapy as adjunctive to surgery and irradiation for treating breast cancer patients. An important issue concerning the proper implementation of these different therapeutic modalities was the timing of the regional therapies (surgery and irradiation) with systemic therapy (chemotherapy.) The type of therapy chosen usually determined the type of subspecialist who would initially see the patient and would dictate the timing of the regional and adjuvant systemic therapies.

Drug dose and dose rate demands for efficacy required that chemotherapy and regional radiation therapy not be given at the same time. If the usual 3-month course of radiation therapy were given immediately following surgery, there were concerns that the time from diagnosis to adjuvant chemotherapy would be too long and would allow the microscopic tumor burden, that the chemotherapy was designed to eliminate, to increase beyond a curable size.

Justification for this concern was first provided by Dr. Cooper's 1969 ASCO abstract (the complete paper was published 10 years later in conjunction with Dr. James Holland). Dr. Cooper reported that his stage II patients with greater than three positive nodes received no benefit from adjuvant CMFVP if it was delayed more than 4 weeks postmastectomy. Those patients who started adjuvant therapy immediately following surgery enjoyed significantly prolonged relapse-free survival.

2.5 LESSONS FROM BASIC SCIENCE

Drs. Howard E. Skipper and Frank M. Shabel, Jr. did pioneering basic science work at the University of Alabama in which they used a mouse model of solid metastatic tumors to study adjuvant chemotherapy. Their studies demonstrated that the incidence of metastases was directly related to the size of the primary cancer. Surgical cure rate of the primary tumor decreased with the rate at which the mass of the tumor increased. If the primary was visible, it was already too large to be cured by chemotherapy. If the drugs used were effective and the primary mass not too large, adjuvant chemotherapy increased the cure of multiple forms of cancer.

They also found in their mouse studies that the stage of similar sized primary cancers was by itself unreliable as a prognostic factor for surgical cure. The timing and the rate of occurrence of metastases were highly variable, so mice with a similar clinical stage had a wide range of microscopic tumor burden. The smaller the tumor burden at surgical excision and the sooner the chemotherapy was begun, the better. Drug or drug combination efficacy, drug dose, and dose rate (with deployment of the most active regimen) were the essential elements necessary for designing a program that could cure microscopic metastatic cancer.

Had these principles been followed earlier in attempts to design successful adjuvant chemotherapy for breast cancer, many lives might have been spared.

Case Study

Sara

Liver Metastases

Sara Dayton was an attractive 43-year-old high school teacher from Houston. In June 1980, she was diagnosed as having a stage I breast cancer in the lower inner quadrant of her left breast. She was diagnosed, staged, and treated at one of the fine medical centers in Houston. Her cancer was small, nodes were negative, and she elected breast conservation surgery followed by radiation therapy. The malignancy was well differentiated and was both estrogen receptor and progesterone receptor positive (ER+ and PR+).

On completing radiation therapy, she began tamoxifen and rapidly resumed her normal active life. She was seen by her medical oncologist every 3–4 months. Her chest X-ray, bone scan, and the carcinoembryonic antigen (CEA) and cancer antigen 15-3 (CA 15-3) serum tumor biomarkers were evaluated annually.

Twelve years after Sara had been diagnosed with breast cancer, the tumor markers started to climb. Shortly thereafter, liver metastases were noted on a computerized tomography (CT) scan. Sara's oncologist advised her that her situation was hopeless and this grim prognosis was seconded by his oncology partner. Neither of these oncologists had observed a meaningful remission with significant extension of life in these circumstances and were attempting to spare Sara the side effects of multiple courses of chemotherapy. But to what advantage?

When the liver lesion was removed, it measured 1.7 cm, so contained far in excess of the 1 billion cells required for visualization. The likelihood was at least 98% that microscopic metastases existed elsewhere in the liver and possibly the bone. But because they were so small, it was not possible to either remove them or to follow their response to radiation or chemotherapy. So the only way Sara could be followed to determine the success of therapy was to observe an absence of recurrence.

The best estimate of the number of cancer cells that could be eliminated by chemotherapy was 1 million cells. Therefore, if a metastasis of 10 million cells were present in the bone marrow when the liver imaging was done, as many as 9 million cells could remain and the bone site would not be cured even though "good" induction adjunct therapy was given. Furthermore, there was no way even to find tumor metastasis in the range between 1 million and 1 billion cells. This was the reason why Blumenschein routinely prescribed radiation to be given to the whole liver and why he was looking for further benefit to be provided by giving a course of consolidation adjuvant chemotherapy after completing the initial induction adjuvant drug therapy. Hopefully, this program would be adequate to tackle the suspected residual tumor burden.

During the 1980s, patients were becoming increasingly assertive in their search for knowledge about available treatment options for their medical problems. Sara, confronted by a situation which seemed hopeless, with the word "cure" never mentioned, asked for her films and records. She planned to scour the country for a physician who could offer at least a modicum of hope and was willing to pursue a yet-to-be-widely-accepted course of action, if it seemed reasonable.

Fortunately, the Susan G. Komen Foundation had been started by Nancy Brinker, a dedicated, highly motivated young woman whose sister, Susan Komen, had died as a result of breast cancer. Nancy, herself, was 2 years postmastectomy and chemotherapy. The Foundation was in its start-up phase in Dallas and its primary goal at that time was to raise funds to support clinical research that would provide a cure of this disease which annually was responsible for the death of more than 40,000 US women during their most productive years. Sara had friends in Dallas who knew Nancy Brinker and Nancy was pleased to meet with her and share her insight about the various breast cancer treatment programs operating in the United States and Europe. She, however, was not aware of a program designed to effect cure as an outcome for patients with metastatic breast cancer, other than the many that were conducting adjuvant trials for stage II disease and were fiercely competing for patients.

At that time, only Blumenschein was attempting to find a cure for stage IV breast cancer. In March 1977, he reported on the treatment of patients who had limited sites of metastatic disease with regional therapy prior to chemoimmunotherapy with FAC and BCG (bacille Calmette Guerin), a vaccine against tuberculosis that was used as an immunostimulant. These patients, who were in complete remission because of surgery or radiation therapy when they started chemotherapy, became known as stage IV NED. In the initial reports, there were no patients with limited and resectable liver metastases, but these were soon included and some had positive outcomes. Nancy was aware of these encouraging results and advised Sara to return to Houston to see Dr. Blumenschein or one of his associates as soon as possible.

This was done. Blumenschein recommended that Sara had the liver lesion completely excised and that surgery should be followed by six courses of the current Adriamycin induction chemotherapy combination: Cytoxan, Adriamycin, and VP-16 (generic name etoposide), abbreviated as CAVe.[1] The most difficult task that confronted Blumenschein was to

---

[1]Etoposide had been substituted for 5-FU at that time because there was a hint that etoposide produced a higher percentage of complete remissions in patients with malignant breast disease than did FAC, but subsequent trials failed to confirm this observation and FAC remained the primary choice for induction adjuvant chemotherapy. This was particularly true for the ACC'91 study of patients with inflammatory breast cancer. Blumenschein regrets that he got locked into CAVe longer than he desired, once he had observed that there was no difference in relapse-free survival and overall survival in FAC-treated patients versus CAVe-treated patients.

find a surgeon willing to perform what would be considered unconventional surgery. Most physicians would expect to find a showering of very small, almost grossly undetectable metastases throughout the liver when the abdomen was opened and the liver visualized. If this were the situation, the surgery would have been futile and inappropriate. Fortunately, percutaneous biopsy of an area of the liver that was away from the site of metastases seen on CT scan was normal, and Dr. Robert Steckler in Dallas agreed to do the surgery. He had recently moved to the "Big D" after completing his surgical oncology training at MDA and was well known and highly respected by the MDA staff.

The resection was clean and the margins were clear of cancer. CAVe was started 10 days after surgery and Sara completed the six 21-day courses over 18 weeks, receiving a total of $300 \, mg/m^2$ of Adriamycin by continuous infusion. Following CAVe, she received three 28-day courses of consolidation adjuvant MCCFUD (methotrexate, cisplatin, 5-FU, and cyclophosphamide with leucovorin rescue). One month following completion of adjuvant chemotherapy, the decision was made to add low-dose late consolidation irradiation to the liver and she received slightly less than 3000 rads. Sara was in complete remission and there was no clinical evidence of cardiac muscle injury. The liver metastases had tested negative for both ER and PR, so tamoxifen was discontinued.

This unexpectedly positive outcome warranted an aggressive follow-up schedule that consisted of a clinical review, physical exam, chest and liver CT, isotope bone scan, and serum tumor markers every 3 months, as well as routine laboratory tests. To everyone's surprise, she remained disease-free at her 24-month visit and these extensive reviews were changed to a 6-month interval. At 5 years when everything was normal, someone switched Sara to an annual follow-up visit, convinced that she was cured.

They were wrong.

In June 2002, 120 months since she began dealing with her first hepatic metastases, her liver CT and her serum CEA level were found to be abnormal. Needle biopsy of the liver lesion again showed metastatic breast cancer. As with many things, however, "time is your friend." When dealing with cancer, this is doubly so. In this case, time was very kind to Sara as it allowed her physicians the opportunity to evaluate a host of compounds and protocols active in other cancers, but never given a critical trial against breast cancer.

After Adriamycin was introduced, there began a search for other chemotherapeutic drugs active against breast cancer and, hopefully, noncross resistant to Adriamycin. In an effort to expand the number of effective therapeutic options, some 2 dozen new chemotherapeutic agents were tested for their activity against breast cancer cells. This, as with many other tasks at MDA, was a joint project between Developmental

Therapeutics and the Medical Breast Service. Dr. Gerald Bodey from Developmental Therapeutics directed the program. Dr. Hwee-Yong Yap from the Medical Breast Service was prodigiously productive in designing and conducting clinical trials of numerous candidate agents.

This massive effort expanded Sara's therapeutic options and Blumenschein could now treat Sara's second liver recurrence with nine courses of a combination of cyclophosphamide, Adriamycin, and taxol (CAT), giving her a cumulative Adriamycin dose of 750 mg/m^2. When the area of liver recurrence was explored surgically after this regimen, multiple biopsies showed no evidence of cancer. So she received a final course of 5-FU, mitomycin C, etoposide, and cisplatin (FUMEP). As of this writing, Sara is doing well without evidence of disease (NED). Accordingly, Blumenschein counts Sara as cured!

CHAPTER 3

The Evolving Goal of Cure and Inflammatory Breast Cancer

Given the current climate of opinion, the initial challenge for a woman who wishes to obtain a cure for an aggressive version of breast cancer that has a poor prognosis is that she needs to identify a medical oncologist who shares her vision of seeking a cure. This physician must be able to outline to her why a new therapeutic regimen might be successful and be willing to discuss the strengths and weaknesses of recommended standard or more popular programs. There should be a reasonable demonstration that the standard or popularly recommended program would result, with time, in death. All real and potential side effects should be clearly explained and the patient must realize she will receive, or may receive, criticism from unexpected sources. A significant period of time should be planned for the initial physician visit, one aspect of which will be for the physician to perceive the patient's depth of understanding. Blumenschein was known for routinely providing his patients with a lengthy initial visit.

3.1 UNDERSTANDING TREATMENT STRATEGY AND THE PERILS OF PROGNOSTICATION

Recently there has been increased interest in end of life issues, particularly with reference to conservation of healthcare funds by not squandering them on hopeless and heroic care. One hears statements by well-meaning, but under-informed, talking heads who claim to be knowledgeable about the prognosis of patients, based on their diagnosis and stage of disease at diagnosis. An example often heard is that we all know that when a patient has a spread of her breast cancer into her liver the situation is hopeless, therefore nothing should be done. This is a dated statement and, as just illustrated by Sara's example, is highly inaccurate.

Blumenschein happened to watch an NBC current events program in which Pat Buchanan was objecting to the thinking that a panel had the wisdom to prognosticate a diagnosis-based outcome for every patient. He qualified this statement by adding that, of course, there were exceptions for which the outcome was inevitable, such as metastatic breast cancer to liver. This comment, given with such certainty, caught Blumenschein's attention and reminded him of a series of breast cancer patients with metastatic disease to the liver that he and Dr. Joseph Kong had treated with induction FAC followed by consolidation MCCFUD chemotherapy and low-dose radiation therapy to the liver. They had treated at least 36 patients, 6 of whom remained free of measurable cancer for more than 30 months after entering remission. Because the sustained remission rate was low (<20%) and the hepatic toxicity caused by the radiation therapy was severe, they lost interest in the project after a year and moved to other clinical treatments. There were other examples of sustained remissions of breast cancer that had metastasized to the liver, but they also were few. Nevertheless, these few successes rendered Buchanan's remark dated and untrue.

However, most people, including physicians, would agree with Buchanan's remark. In fact, one of the events that motivated the author to begin planning this book was a discussion about "death panels," and their place in containing the rise in healthcare costs. This discussion was being carried out with insufficient appreciation that the ability to make accurate prognostic assessments requires intimate familiarity with current aggressive treatments that work. Decisions of this magnitude require up-to-the-minute knowledge about all variations of each disease and the status of ongoing research and current new treatment attempts. Only then can patients and families be truly informed.

For example, to have a cancer that is ER+ has always been considered good, while ER− cancers were considered bad. However, chemotherapy drugs and drug combinations now exist that can kill every last breast cancer cell. So the more rapidly growing clinically aggressive ER− cancer cells are the first to be killed. As a result, the "bad" cancers regress more rapidly than the "good," illustrating one of Freireich's dictums that "the bad is good and the good is bad." Fortunately, there is an additional therapeutic maneuver that can be used in ER+ and PR+ breast cancers. These cells can be killed or placed in division arrest by removing the organ of estrogen production, the ovaries, or by blocking estrogen access to its cellular receptors using a drug like tamoxifen in premenopausal women. In postmenopausal women, an aromatase inhibitor is used to block the formation of estrogen from androgens that are formed in peripheral tissues.

A definition of complete remission would be that through therapy (surgery, irradiation, and/or chemotherapy), there occurs a complete elimination of every measurable focus of cancer cells in the body. Complete remission can be described for the entire patient or for separate organs. For example, a patient with liver metastasis from her breast cancer would be described as having stage IV breast cancer with liver metastases. If the liver lesions disappear as a result of therapy, she remains stage IV in complete remission with a liver in complete remission.

If the cancer is ER− and no further therapy is given, after 3 years, the patient may begin to consider herself cured. However, if maintenance therapy of any sort is used to support the complete remission, then 5 years posttherapy is required to gain a level of comfort with a designation of cure. For example, if the cancer is ER+ and the patient maintains the complete remission while taking tamoxifen for 5 years, then in most cases 10 years have to pass before she can truly consider herself cured. However, in each instance complete remission is the gateway to cure.

3.2 INFLAMMATORY BREAST CANCER

Inflammatory breast cancer (IBC) has a particularly feared reputation as a form of cancer that is diagnosed when a patient presents to her physician after rapid development of a warm, erythematous, and swollen breast. The diagnosis can be made clinically but is unequivocal when histological examination shows dermal lymphatics containing sheets of cancer cells. Prior to the advent of effective chemotherapy, the prognosis of patients with this diagnosis was similar to that of an aggressive stage IV primary that was locally advanced and did not respond to any form of therapy. Most patients died within 2 years. Surgeons refused to do mastectomies because skin metastases would begin to appear on the chest wall even before wound healing was complete. The remaining therapeutic option was radiation therapy, which did a superb job in containing tumor growth in the breast but was ineffective against systemic disease. Fortunately, the occurrence of IBC was rare, showing up in only about 3−6% of newly diagnosed patients.

The majority of IBC cells are ER−, are very homogenous in their behavior, and usually express their uniformity early. In this respect IBC is an excellent, but unfortunate, expression of breast cancer. An example of the similarity of outcomes in IBC can be seen in two trials (MDA'94 and ACC'91) that compare relapse-free survival. For example, if a patient relapsed, it occurred very close to 11 months. This made the population of patients with IBC an excellent group for "proof of concept" trials that were then used to guide subsequent longer studies with larger patient groups. The problem was, if the results of an initial proof of concept study were unequivocal, it subsequently became difficult to treat patients with programs that were obviously inferior.

If the clinical behavior of IBC was very aggressive, its response to FAC or CAVe was equally dramatic in proof of concept trials. Ninety percent of these patients had such an extensive immediate response to the Adriamycin combinations that it was decided to have patients undergo a debulking mastectomy just prior to the time when they would be normally starting their fourth course of chemotherapy. Three weeks postmastectomy, radiation therapy was begun to the chest wall and the peripheral lymph nodes on the side of the mastectomy. The radiation therapy was given over 6 weeks and an additional 3 weeks were required for normal tissue recovery. While overall survival was extended, every patient in this initial IBC group eventually died with widespread metastatic breast cancer.

It was immediately clear where the problem lay: the break in the dose rate of chemotherapy required for the surgery and radiation therapy gave the cancer a 12-week respite from chemotherapy. Thus, the tens and hundreds of millions of cancer cells outside the radiation fields that were dying from the initial three courses of chemotherapy and radiation had time to recover, multiply and mutate, and reappear as drug-resistant metastases.

This realization resulted in revision of the IBC treatment protocol. The induction Adriamycin combination, CAVe, was changed so that it was given every 3 weeks ×6, with the debulking mastectomy in responding patients following the third course of CAVe. This created the difficulty of combining mastectomy with the neutropenia that accompanied the CAVe. But the oncologists quickly learned that, with appropriate wound care and aggressive antibiotic therapy, they could maneuver their patients through the complex third course of CAVe that was usually started on day 2 or 3 after surgery. Learning to simultaneously deliver chemotherapy and reduce visible metastases surgically allowed more strict protocol adherence to the dose-rate requirements of chemotherapy. So CAVe or FAC ×6, with mastectomy as part of the third course, followed by MCCFUD ×3, and concluding with radiation therapy became the MDA and subsequent ACC protocol for treatment of IBC.

After two patients were so treated in a proof of concept trial and remained relapse free beyond 2 years, Blumenschein began to enter all IBC patients on this altered program. The only difficulty he encountered was the length of the interval between CAVe cycles 3 and 4. The majority of the patients had a 28-day interval after surgery rather than the prescribed 21 days.

3.3 THE SEARCH FOR NEW DRUGS TO CURE IBC

Very early in the follow-up of IBC patients, it became evident that there would be a place for a non-cross-resistant chemotherapy regimen to be given as consolidation adjuvant therapy to patients in complete remission after they had completed induction adjuvant treatment. Blumenschein was interested in validating a role for consolidation adjuvant chemotherapy to achieve cures in patients whose breast cancer had a poor prognosis. However, the Medical Breast Service at MDA initially lacked an effective combination chemotherapy regimen which was non-cross-resistant to FAC and could be employed as a consolidation adjuvant therapy. A lack of cross-resistance was necessary in order to justify the inclusion of this additional drug therapy in consolidation regimens that might achieve lasting complete remissions.

There was a momentary bright spot in establishing the proof for this concept when Dr. Aman Buzdar and Dr. Gabriel Hortobagyi published a clinical trial in which they showed that the combination of methotrexate and Velban (vinblastine) (MTX/VLB) might fulfill that need when given in the consolidation setting to ER+ stage II breast cancer patients who had been previously treated with mastectomy, six courses of FAC, and tamoxifen. On completing FAC, and while continuing tamoxifen, every other patient was assigned to 8-day cycles of MTX/VLB. After 2 years, Buzdar and Hortobagyi found that the

MTX/VLB treated patients had a superior relapse-free survival that was statistically significant.

Unfortunately, there were many uncomfortable issues in the conduct of the trial, and there was an even larger question as to whether one could consider MTX/VLB to be late-consolidation chemotherapy because of the schedule of administration. Blumenschein was against giving it this designation because survival was prolonged in only 35% of patients with FAC-treated cancers who received this drug combination. Fortunately, several more promising drugs became available that could be included in combination therapy regimens.

3.4 MCCFUD AND FUMEP FOR IBC

Cisplatin (CDDP) was long known to be an active agent for the treatment of breast cancer. It, however, was an inconvenient drug, being associated with severe nausea, impaired renal function, and protracted and significant thrombocytopenia. After observing the excellent response of a breast cancer patient with liver metastases who was inadvertently treated with single-agent CDDP, Blumenschein felt that a place could be found for the drug in a combination that would qualify as the long-sought consolidation adjuvant program.

So during the late 1970s and early 1980s, Blumenschein evaluated several CDDP combinations and eventually selected a drug combination of methotrexate with leucovorin rescue, CDDP, cyclophosphamide, and 5-FU (MCCFUD). He gauged the relative activity of MCCFUD consolidation therapy by measuring the antitumor response to the drug combination in breast cancers that had been treated previously with FAC and CMF induction therapy. As shown in Table 3.1,

Table 3.1 Response to MCCFUD Consolidation Therapy Based on Response to Induction Therapy	
Induction Scenario	**MCCFUD Response Rate (%)**
Prior FAC induction	67
If responsive to FAC	75
If unresponsive to FAC	30
Prior CMF induction	43
If responsive to CMF	67

Presented by Blumenschein GR, Wagner K, Hanks S, Dieke KA at the Eighth Annual Multidisciplinary Symposium on Breast Disease, University of Florida, Amelia Island, FL, February 13–16, 2003.

the 67% response rate to MCCFUD in the 66 metastatic breast cancer patients initially treated with FAC fulfilled the requirements for a late-consolidation adjuvant program, and results were even more convincing in those patients who had been responsive to FAC therapy.

So the ACC developed a protocol for IBC patients to establish evidence that the limited addition of three courses of consolidation MCCFUD at the conclusion of FAC induction chemotherapy would result in an increase of cures. In 1985, the induction chemotherapy was switched from FAC to CAVe and a total of 71 patients were enrolled in three sequential clinical trials that were conducted over 14 years (ACC'91, A, B, C) (Table 3.2). Thus, three protocols were used by Blumenschein to treat IBC from January 1985 to July 1999. Over the initial 6 years from January 1985 to January 1991, patient accrual was slow, but by staying with the IBC protocol that used six courses of the most efficacious Adriamycin-based induction adjuvant program with mastectomy after the third course and cross over to the most active, non-cross-resistant late-consolidation chemotherapy following the sixth course of CAVe, he was able to accrue 23 IBC patients.

Table 3.2 Summary of ACC'91 Trial in 71 Patients with IBC[*]			
	Group A	Group B	Group C
Treatment dates	1/85–1/91	2/91–11/96	12/96–7/99
Number of patients	23	33	15
Induction regimen	CAVe	CAVe	CAT
Consolidation regimen	MCCFUD	FUMEP	FUMEP
Follow-up time (months)	144–216	74–140	42–72
% Disease free	65%	61%	73%

[*]Presented by Blumenschein GR, Wagner K, Hanks S, Dieke KA at the Eighth Annual Multidisciplinary Symposium on Breast Disease, University of Florida, Amelia Island, FL, February 13–16, 2003.

A new four-drug regimen that consisted of 5-FU, mitomycin C, etoposide, and cisplatin (FUMEP) was developed which Blumenschein believed from his clinical trials was superior to MCCFUD. So the adjuvant consolidation protocol was switched from MCCFUD to FUMEP in February 1991. During the next 5½ years, 33 newly diagnosed IBC patients were entered on this new protocol. However, this regimen contained two unattractive drugs: mitomycin C and cisplatin. Mitomycin in particular had dose-limiting toxicity that was appropriately named the "hemolytic–uremic" syndrome. This syndrome is fatal if not dealt with appropriately and is characterized by a rapid onset of red blood cell lysis and attendant anemia, decreased blood platelet count, and acute renal failure.

3.5 TAXANES

Taxanes entered the arena with reports of impressive overall remission rates in treating patients with metastatic breast cancer. Two of these regimens, CAT (cyclophosphamide, Adriamycin, and taxol) and TAC (taxotere, Adriamycin, and cyclophosphamide) had raised the overall remission rate to 91–94%, with complete remissions of 32% in metastatic breast cancer patients. However, there remained a question for some time: Which was better, taxol or taxotere? The general consensus by the early 1990s had placed taxotere and TAC in the winner's circle.

Based on these improved remission rates, Blumenschein in December 1996 replaced the FAC induction adjuvant protocol with 6 courses of CAT and an additional 15 IBC patients came into the study and received this more effective regimen during the final accrual period. The response to CAVe in the 23 patients in group A had been sufficient to allow mastectomy to place each patient in complete remission and similar results were obtained in the 33 patients in group B. However, while the 15 patients who were treated with CAT in group C were too few for statistical significance to be established, the percentage of Group C patients relapsing by 36 months was only 27%, as compared to 35% in Group A and 39% in Group B (Table 3.2). Not only did CAT induction appear to put a larger proportion of IBC patients into complete remission but the 73% of Group C patients who were disease free at 6 years strongly suggested that switching the induction adjuvant regimen from FAC or CAVe to CAT was beneficial.

3.6 COMBINATION CHEMOTHERAPY VERSUS MONOTHERAPY FOR CONSOLIDATION REGIMENS

In a final analysis, the results of these three separate proof of concept studies were put together as a single trial (ACC'91), principally to assess the value of late-consolidation adjuvant chemotherapy for achieving long-term complete remissions and cure in a primary form of breast cancer that prior to 1985 was considered equivalent to stage

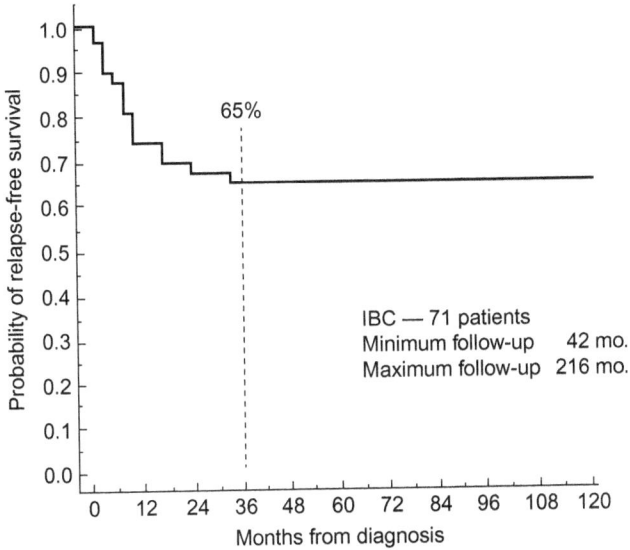

Figure 3.1 Kaplan−Meier survival curve for the 71 IBC patients that were combined in ACC'91 to analyze the efficacy of consolidation chemotherapy. By 3 years, survival had reached a plateau of 65%. (Presented by Blumenschein GR, Wagner K, Hanks S, Dieke KA at the 8th Annual Multidisciplinary Symposium on Breast Disease, University of Florida, Amelia Island, FL, February 13–16, 2003.)

IV disease. The overall response of these patients is illustrated by the Kaplan−Meier survival curve shown in Figure 3.1 and supports the concept that a brief program of consolidation therapy can enhance outcomes in these patients.

When taxanes became available, the Medical Breast Service at MDA also was impressed with taxol's activity in patients with breast cancer and thought it would be a good consolidation drug as a single agent following induction adjuvant for IBC treatment. Therefore, in 1994 the Medical Breast Service at MDA launched a new consolidation protocol (MDA'94) in which, following FAC induction adjuvant therapy, taxol was used as a single agent for consolidation chemotherapy of IBC patients. Thus, the ACC'91 protocol that incorporated MCCFUD or FUMEP as consolidation therapy in Groups A, B, and C was able to compare its outcome to a very similar but different program. Because the induction chemotherapy regimen was similar in the two protocols, the major difference between them was the use of taxol as a consolidation single agent in the MDA'94 protocol instead of MCCFUD or FUMEP in ACC'91. It was found that the percentage of patients in the MDA'94 program who were disease free at 2 years was 58% and was 49% at 3 years, whereas somewhat better outcomes were achieved in ACC'91 group of trials (Figure 3.1). Although it was difficult to obtain exact 5-year and 10-year relapse-free survival data from the MDA'94 trial, it was clear that the patients who were in histologic complete remission and had the best prognosis, had a relapse-free survival of 38% that plateaued at around 4–5 years and remained so at 10 years.

There has been only one relapse beyond 10 years in the ACC'91 group of IBC patients who obtained a long-term complete remission. This occurred 11 years post diagnosis and treatment of IBC in a 47-year-old patient whose cancer was ER + but who had never received tamoxifen. Prior to this, Blumenschein believed that if an ER+ patient remained in complete remission off therapy for more than 7 years, she was cured. Needless to say, his treatment protocol for ER+ IBC patients was modified to include indefinite administration of tamoxifen. A second ER+ IBC patient, on long-term follow-up but not in the ACC'91 study, relapsed 26 years after initial diagnosis with a cancer in the same breast as the original occurrence. She had completed the six FAC courses, radiation therapy, and six courses of MCCFUD, but had refused mastectomy. Unfortunately, tamoxifen was never considered. Had she started tamoxifen 26 years ago and continued to the present, she might continue to be in tamoxifen-sustained complete remission.

Regrettably, comparable studies attempting to assess modifications in existing regimens and their effect on outcome were not as focused on the concept of consolidation adjuvant chemotherapy as a means of eradicating minimal residual tumor that remained after induction adjuvant therapy. Instead, these studies addressed questions, such as: What will be the impact of 5-FU on the complete response and partial response of the FAC program? Will the current use of only Adriamycin and cyclophosphamide (AC) be of lesser activity than FAC? Never asked were more important questions, such as "Can this be cured at this stage? If so, how?"

If these were the first questions asked, wouldn't asking them have improved the focus of the research?

Case Study

Martha

The Texas Challenge

Martha, age 26, was an attractive and busy mother of three preschool children. Her husband Michael, a successful banker, was active in community and church affairs. While not directly involved in politics, they did live in Austin and, as alumni of the University of Texas, kept current in knowing what was significant in their great state of Texas. In April 1974, that would have included the cognizance that if a person had to deal with the dreaded diagnosis of cancer, there was no greater institution than MDA for diagnosis, staging, and treatment of cancer in Texas, the United States, and, indeed, the world. At the time, MDA was one of two comprehensive cancer centers in the United States and it was part of the University of Texas. One could with confidence receive state-of-the-art care for any of the multiple expressions of cancer.

Unfortunately, in April 1974, Martha found a mass in her left breast. The following morning, Michael canceled his meetings, bundled their three children off to his in-laws, and took Martha to a general surgeon, Dr. Parker, who had insisted he see her immediately when Michael phoned. Dr. Parker confirmed the presence of a 4-cm mass in the upper outer quadrant of Martha's left breast and palpated enlarged lymph nodes in her left axilla. Within 72 h, a mammogram and ultrasound confirmed the physical examination, and a core needle biopsy was scheduled. The biopsy was read as a poorly differentiated ductal adenocarcinoma of the breast. Dr. Parker recommended that Martha undergo a modified radical mastectomy as her initial therapy.

Martha and Michael had a host of questions. They asked for details about the surgery. Were there complications to be expected? Was this the only surgical approach that would be considered? What were the chances this therapeutic approach would result in a cure? Here the surgeon paused, and in a careful and measured tone responded, "The answer to that question will depend on your stage of cancer. Your stage, to a great degree, will be determined by the number of axillary lymph nodes found to contain metastatic cancer. Currently, I consider you to have stage II breast cancer. I would prefer to reserve further discussion of this question until I have more details."

In 1974, it was uncommon for a physician to enter into a lengthy and detailed discussion of the probable outcome of the treatment of a serious illness, especially when it was considered to be negative. This information was transmitted to the patient gradually by contacts and discussions with her physician, other physicians, nurses, other patients, periodicals, and newspapers. Dr. Parker was pressed for time. He had worked Martha into his busy schedule as a favor to an associate and felt further discourse was unnecessary. His impression of the situation was that Martha had multiple nodes involved with metastatic cancer and a poor prognosis. Before Parker could leave, however, Michael had one additional question: Would Parker refer Martha to MDA for a second opinion?

This is the most delicate question a patient can ask a physician. It contains the implication that there may be another, more knowledgeable and experienced doctor who might better serve the patient, resulting in the transfer of care to the consultant with the location of this care at a different site. The concern about loss of cancer patients to MDA by physicians in the Houston area was such that the average distance from MDA to its patients was 150 miles. Fortunately, Dr. Parker had no ego problems and, in fact, looked forward to the recommendation he would receive. He phoned his good friend, Dr. Richard Martin, Chief of Surgery at MDA, and asked him to see Martha as soon as possible. Upon her arrival at the MDA registration office, Martha was met by Doris, a VIP patient care representative, whose job was to smooth any potential rough spots before they became an issue. After discussion with Dr. Parker, Dr. Martin scheduled a bone scan and an isotope liver scan in order to complete her preoperative staging prior to her initial visit with him.

In 1974, the standard approach in treating patients with advanced primary breast cancer was to perform a modified radical mastectomy which removed the cancer, the breast, and the axillary lymph nodes draining the involved breast. When nodes were involved, radiation therapy was begun about 3 weeks after surgery to allow the surgical wound to heal. At this time, there was a great deal of clinical research being conducted to establish the place for chemotherapy in the treatment spectrum of patients with advanced primary breast cancer. Clinically, Martha was stage IIB and would be a candidate for chemotherapy after completing radiation therapy. The issue was going to be what type of chemotherapy. However, the direction that Martha's postoperative therapy was going to take was suddenly dictated by events. As Doris took her to radiology for the radioisotope injection prior to the bone scan, Martha had a grand mal seizure. Dr. Martin was notified, and he asked Dr. Blumenschein, recently appointed Head of the Medical Breast Service, to assume her management.

There was no history of seizure in Martha's past and her brain scan was unremarkable. She was admitted to the hospital for observation, a spinal tap, and an electroencephalogram (EEG). While no evidence for a brain metastasis could be found, it was assumed that was the cause of her seizure. Because there was no detectable brain lesion on which surgery or radiation therapy could focus, it was decided that chemotherapy might offer some benefit, if it crossed the blood–brain barrier. However, for purposes of tumor debulking and staging, she first needed to undergo a left modified radical mastectomy, to include an axillary dissection on the left. Technically, she would remain in stage IIB unless regional spread of cancer or under-measurement of tumor size was discovered at surgery and/or measurable brain metastases appeared.

Understandably, Martha and Michael had been quite shaken by the rapid turn of events, but realized that the best course was to push on as aggressively as possible. They were informed that, because of the concern about her seizure, radiation therapy was not to follow surgery, as was usual. Rather, chemotherapy consisting of at least six courses of FAC would be started 2 weeks after her mastectomy.

The surgery and pathology examination established that Martha had a 4 cm tumor and 18 axillary lymph nodes involved with metastatic breast cancer. Her stage remained the same, IIB, but her prognosis grew worse as a result of the 18 positive lymph nodes. Without effective adjuvant chemotherapy, Martha had less than a 50% chance of remaining disease free beyond 2 years from diagnosis and a 12% chance for survival after 10 years. This meant that at diagnosis she had a >88% probability of harboring lethal microscopic metastatic breast cancer. This gave Martha a prognosis approaching that of patients with stage IV breast cancer and raised a question about the clinical wisdom of treating her with anything less than the most aggressive drug program then available for patients with metastatic breast cancer.

Fortunately, Dr. Buzdar had initiated MDA's adjuvant chemotherapy program for postmastectomy stage II patients with positive nodes and stage III breast cancer in January 1974. So in April, Martha began FAC 2 weeks after her mastectomy. At this same time, competing investigator teams around the world were beginning to address this issue with less aggressive combination chemotherapy programs, such as CMF (Dr. Bonadonna in Milan), L-PAM—5-FU (Dr. Bernard Fisher, NSABP, in Pittsburgh), and AC (Drs. Stephen E. Jones and Sydney E. Salmon in Arizona).

Toxicity was never a significant factor for Martha during her program of FAC administration. That is to say, toxicity never was severe enough to cause a lowering of a drug dose or a prolongation of a treatment interval (dose rate). She experienced nausea, occasional vomiting, mucositis, and 100% hair loss, but there were no EKG changes. One episode of temperature elevation also occurred during a time when her white blood cells were depleted and caused her to be hospitalized to receive IV antibiotic therapy. Martha's experience was typical of most patients who received FAC in that adjustments and minor modifications in the toxicity protocols were able to solve most issues. Those that remained eventually fell to the magic of outpatient pump technology that permitted continuous-infusion Adriamycin administration, which minimized myocardial toxicity, and Neupogen (granulocyte colony stimulating factor), which bolstered production of white blood cells.

When the FAC protocol was initially designed, concerns about the persistence of a reduced but still viable microscopic tumor burden led to prolonged maintenance chemotherapy of patients who had completed 6 months of FAC induction chemotherapy. In the MDA FAC program, this consisted of CMF cycles that were given on a monthly schedule for 18 months after induction adjuvant therapy. The CMF regimen was given intramuscularly and by mouth, as a patient's veins were thoroughly trashed after 6 months of FAC. The dose and schedule of each of the drugs was as follows: cyclophosphamide 500 mg/m^2 orally in four divided doses on day 2 of each 28-day cycle, methotrexate 30 mg/m^2 intramuscularly on days 1 and 8, and 5-FU 500 mg/m^2 orally in 4 divided doses on days 1 and 8.

To further complicate the situation, it was decided that patients should not be denied the possible benefits of immunotherapy, so BCG was added to the program (6×10^8 viable units of the Connaught strain given by scarification on days 9, 16, and 23 of each cycle). Immunotherapy was part of a rigid belief system and BCG was its trinity. Emotions ran high every time it was discussed. To his discredit, Blumenschein supported its inclusion in the MDA adjuvant breast protocol. However, he began to worry about his judgment when one of the proponents of BCG was heard to challenge an opponent by asking, "Would you deny your mother BCG?"

The scarifications, aptly named, were visible and permanent. In a notable episode, an attractive young breast cancer patient on the BCG protocol was taking a stroll on a Florida beach. It wasn't very long before she acquired an ardent male admirer. He became overly persistent in asking too many questions. She put an end to things when she answered his query as to the reason for the multiple scars on her upper arms, thighs, and shoulders. "Don't be concerned," she said, "it's a new treatment for syphilis."

Martha made it through the first 12 months without missing a beat, but her enthusiasm began to wane as she contemplated a second 12 months of CMF and BCG. Her oncologists also began to realize that the CMF maintenance dose, schedule, and route of administration were inferior. Even the concept was inferior if the goal of the chemotherapy, indeed, was cure. With the BCG component, patients began to suffer from "scarification burn out." Suffice it to say, all of the patients continued to receive full doses of FAC. The other elements of the program were given and received with less enthusiasm and diligence.

For a comparative evaluation of the FAC protocol, a group of stage II and III breast cancer patients with at least one involved axillary node, who were treated at MDA with surgery and/or radiation therapy with curative intent, were selected for close follow-up in a study that utilized historical controls. After examining the records of patients treated between January 1972 and December 1973, 152 patients were found who were similar enough to the FAC-treated patients to qualify for the historical control group. The only subset of patients that was not evenly matched between the groups was the group with >10 positive lymph nodes. Because 40% of the patients in the FAC-treated group had >10 positive nodes while only 25% of controls were so staged, the control group was expected to have a slight survival advantage. However, an initial analysis at 1-year postmastectomy showed that 94% of the FAC–BCG patients remained relapse free whereas only 75% of the control patients had been disease free. At 2 years, the relapse-free outcomes were 93 and 55%, respectively. Thus, the study showed conclusively that the FAC adjuvant program benefited pre- and postmenopausal, stage II and III breast cancer patients. Although Martha had >10 positive nodes, she was indeed fortunate to have developed her breast cancer at a time when she could be placed in the FAC treatment group!

Irradiation is an effective killer of breast cancer cells and plays an important role in eliminating microscopic metastases from the chest wall and peripheral lymphatics on the side of the mastectomy. It is an established therapeutic modality for the adjuvant treatment of node-positive disease. However, there are some limitations in its use. The time required to deliver a therapeutic dose of ionizing irradiation is usually 5–6 weeks, which is delivered daily Monday through Friday. During this time, concomitant Adriamycin chemotherapy should be avoided and there should always be a 3-week interval between radiation and Adriamycin therapy. Because of the daily schedule required for radiation therapy, Martha chose to receive her radiation therapy in Austin. It began 4 weeks after her sixth and final course of FAC.

Martha had no further problem with seizures but she was fatigued and worn down from the 6 months of therapy. Fortunately, there was no sign of heart muscle damage even though she had received a total of 240 mg/m^2 of Adriamycin, still given at that time by IV bolus. While she did begin the maintenance program after the radiation therapy and continued to receive CMF and BCG for the first 12 months period following diagnosis, mutual enthusiasm to continue beyond 15 months was lacking and her adjuvant therapy was discontinued. This seemed reasonable because it had been noted in other programs by this time that the results after 12 months of adjuvant treatment were no different than those achieved after 24 months. In fact, BCG as adjuvant and CMF as maintenance therapy have never been shown in a clinical trial to influence patient outcome.

Martha was seen by Blumenschein at 3-month intervals for the first 10 years after diagnosis, at which time she graduated to an annual visit. Currently, she continues to remain free of breast cancer 36 years following regional therapy with a modified radical mastectomy, radiation therapy, and systemic therapy with FAC induction followed by BCG and CMF maintenance.

This more than likely qualifies as a cure!

CHAPTER 4

Adjuvant Therapy Advances

The initial attempt to include chemotherapy as an adjuvant to surgery in treating patients with breast cancer occurred in 1958. It consisted of an NSABP trial to measure the impact of perioperative thiotepa on relapse-free and overall survival of patients with node-positive breast cancer who were undergoing a radical mastectomy. A second early adjuvant study was conducted by Roar Nissen-Meyer in Norway in 1965. He evaluated the effect of perioperative cyclophosphamide on the survival of patients with node-positive breast cancer. Though results were minimally positive in premenopausal women with one to three positive nodes, these trials did not generate a great deal of enthusiasm. In fact, the *perioperative* delivery of adjuvant chemotherapy was fundamentally flawed because it was based on the misconception that metastases occurred when small clumps of tumor cells were released from the breast into the circulation during mastectomy.

The fact that most primary breast cancers would be considered large and probably metastatic when diagnosed began to be appreciated in the 1960s as understanding grew that Skipper and Shabel's observations of the quantitative and qualitative cellular factors that were associated with the development of cancer metastases in mice were also applicable to human malignancies. If cure was the goal of adjuvant chemotherapy, then attention needed to focus on the efficacy of drugs and especially on drug combinations. Unfortunately, large numbers of breast cancer patients who had generously participated in clinical trials received lackluster therapies in less than optimum doses. In the worst case, they received just a placebo and only served as controls to determine if cancer survival could be improved in the group of patients who actually received the experimental chemotherapy.

Combination drug programs started to be explored in the mid-1960s. In 1966, Dr. Ezra M. Greenspan, from Mt. Sinai in New York City, reported increased responses to combination chemotherapy in patients with advanced stage IV breast cancer. This was followed by Dr. Richard Cooper's exciting report of a 68% response in metastatic breast cancer from CMFVP at the 1969 ASCO meeting. Blumenschein, then a fellow in hematology at Duke, was nearly fired because of his use of CMFVP. He treated a private patient of the Chief of Hematology with CMFVP without getting permission from the Chief, who believed in single agent chemotherapy when treating breast cancer. Paradoxically, the Chief was attempting at the same time to explain why patients with Hodgkin's Disease do so poorly when treated with single agent procarbazine, whereas those treated with MOPP (combination of Mustargen, Oncovin, procarbazine, and prednisone) did much better. Fortunately, the metastatic breast cancer patient in question, who had never responded to a host of single agents, responded to the CMFVP. There was no evidence, however, that this had any impact on the Chief's bias against using combination drug therapy to treat patients with breast cancer!

In the early 1970s, many effective combination regimens emerged that were directed at specific tumor types and gave medical oncology the necessary impetus it needed to be recognized as a medical subspecialty. In 1973, Dr. Bonadonna, who had refined CMFVP into CMF, began a series of adjuvant trials in postoperative patients in Milan. He was evaluating the impact of treatment duration, 6 months versus 12, on relapse-free and overall survival. Issues of drug dose, dose rate, and the use of active drugs in sequence versus concurrent use were explored and defined.

In 1974, Dr. Aman Buzdar began the MDA breast cancer adjuvant trial with FAC. At the time, there was only one other adjuvant drug combination trial that included Adriamycin. In this trial, Drs. Salmon and Jones at the Arizona Cancer Center combined IV bolus Adriamycin 30 mg/m^2 with oral cyclophosphamide, to begin postoperatively and continue for 6 months in node-positive patients. The MDA program differed from the others in that the use of adjuvant radiation therapy had been limited in other adjuvant chemotherapy trials. However, since all patients entered in the MDA study were node-positive, they also received radiation therapy. This was given postmastectomy over 6 weeks and required a 3-week interval between the last dose of radiation therapy and the initiation of FAC. These patients, therefore, had an almost 3-month delay from removal of their primary tumor to the start of chemotherapy. Eventually, the adverse effect of this long delay was demonstrated conclusively in Cooper's 1979 report on the adjuvant use of CMFVP.

By 1976, the results of some of these adjuvant trials began to materialize. Dr. Bonadonna's Milan trial showed that CMF was beneficial for premenopausal patients with one to three positive nodes. At MDA, both pre- and postmenopausal breast cancer patients with positive nodes had an increased relapse-free survival from FAC. Their physicians were very impressed by the activity of this program and felt that FAC had proven itself to be the standard against which all other chemotherapy regimens should be measured. So as CMF was considered to be less effective for adjuvant treatment of patients with stage I breast cancer, it was replaced at MDA by FAC.

4.1 PREPARED MINDS TAKE ON BREAST CANCER

As its reputation grew, the Medical Breast Service became a much-sought-after location in which to launch an oncology career. Blumenschein was confronted by an embarrassment of riches in the number of very intelligent, motivated, young physicians who wanted to build their career around the study of breast cancer. Fortunately, the increase in breast cancer patients coming to MDA and the institution's interest in this malignancy allowed many of these superb individuals to join the Medical Breast Service and further their pursuit of knowledge about this disorder.

Dr. Buzdar chose the task of shepherding the all-important adjuvant therapy issues that arose. Dr. Gabriel Hortogabyi took on the responsibility for new drug development, plus anything else he felt would be important. Through his own work and his close and helpful supervision of medical oncology fellows, he was responsible for seminal observations about prognostic factors in breast cancer and the radiographic changes associated with the healing of lytic bone metastases. Drs. Hwee-Yong Yap, Sewa Legha, Robert Benjamin, and Alfred DiStefano rounded out an exceptional team of physician researchers who established the outstanding reputation of the MDA Medical Breast Service.

Dr. Yap discovered that vinblastine, when given IV by continuous infusion, was about three times more active than if the same dose were given as a bolus injection. Thus, in a patient with metastatic breast cancer, vinblastine given in a dose of 10 mg/m^2 IV every 2 weeks would give a partial response about 8% of the time. If the same dose was given by continuous infusion, 2.0 mg/m^2 over 24 h for 5 days every 2 weeks, 30% of the patients could expect at least a partial remission.

4.2 MINIMIZING ADRIAMYCIN CARDIAC TOXICITY: THE MOST SIGNIFICANT UNDER-UTILIZED CLINICAL OBSERVATION

Dr. Yap's seminal observation prompted a re-evaluation of the schedule being used for the administration of all of the significant chemotherapy drugs in use at that time. Adriamycin, of course, was one such drug. No one was certain which fellow made the observation that the EKGs of patients receiving Adriamycin 50 mg/m^2 by continuous infusion over 96 h showed less decrease in QRS voltage, the electrical signal that accompanies contraction of ventricular heart muscle, than did the EKGs taken after a similar cumulative dose of the drug was given by IV bolus.

Dr. Legha, who was on loan to the Medical Breast Service from Dr. Freireich's group, saw the value in this observation and organized a study to determine if heart muscle damage from cumulative Adriamycin could be controlled by modifying the drug administration schedule. Eleven patients were studied who were receiving Adriamycin by continuous infusion. Adriamycin was infused over 48–96 h every 3 weeks at a dose of 60 mg/m^2 until a cumulative Adriamycin dose of 200–250 mg/m^2 was reached. At that point, cardiac muscle biopsies were obtained and were examined by electron microscopy to quantify myocardial damage, scored on a scale of 0–4 with grade 4 being the worst. As long as the patients were responding and there was no evidence of cardiomyopathy, Adriamycin was continued. The biopsies were repeated at 420–480 mg/m^2 cumulative dose and continued at 200–250 mg/m^2 dose increments.

One of the 11 patients reached grade 3 cardiac toxicity at a 480 mg/m^2 cumulative Adriamycin dose and a second reached grade 2 at a 780 mg/m^2 cumulative dose. Adriamycin was discontinued in both. These two patients each had also had 5000 rads of precordial irradiation that may have contributed to this toxicity. On the other hand, there was no evidence of myocardial damage in the nine patients who had received a median Adriamycin dose of 630 mg/m^2 (range: 360–1500 mg/m^2). This ability of continuous infusion to decrease the risk of myocardial damage and subsequent heart failure caused by Adriamycin was confirmed by

Drs. Ewer, Benjamin, and Legha. Because of this observation and its confirmation, we concluded that the cardiac toxicity of Adriamycin was related to its peak concentration in plasma. So after 1979, it was administered only by continuous infusion on the Medical Breast Service. Minimizing the risk of heart failure from the use of Adriamycin, allowed it to be given in situations in which, heretofore, it could not be considered. For example, concern for its cardiac toxicity had previously limited cumulative Adriamycin doses to $450-500 \, mg/m^2$ when bolus doses were administered. Beyond this cumulative dose, heart damage was all too common.

When patients with metastatic breast cancer were treated with FAC, the remission rate at $30 \, mg/m^2$ Adriamycin per course was 40%, at $40 \, mg/m^2$ was 60%, at $50 \, mg/m^2$ was 75%, and at $60 \, mg/m^2$ was 75%. So maximal therapeutic responses were reached when the Adriamycin dose given in FAC was $50-55 \, mg/m^2$ per course. There also was a clear plateau in the slope of the cumulative dose-response curve at a cumulative dose of $400 \, mg/m^2$. This made escalation of Adriamycin dosage beyond that level unnecessary, because it would confer no further benefit and only add additional toxicity.

The timing of successive treatment cycles, which determined dose rate, also appeared to be important, especially when higher Adriamycin doses were administered. Optimal tumor response and bone marrow recovery seems to have been obtained with a 21-day treatment interval. Because further tumor regression would not be seen after the eighth cycle of FAC, it wasn't necessary to treat beyond a $400 \, mg/m^2$ cumulative Adriamycin dose.

So if the goal was to cure breast cancer with chemotherapy, both drug dose and cycle timing had to be chosen with great care.

4.3 CLINICAL MEASUREMENTS: PREDICTING PROGNOSIS

Most of the knowledge and insight the MDA medical oncologists gained about breast cancer and FAC was from the very thorough assessment of clinical information gathered from the initial group of 619 stage IV breast cancer patients with previously untreated metastatic breast cancer. All these patients received some version of FAC as initial therapy and were then continued on to BCG-CMF in an attempt to see if there was any value or issue with this maintenance therapy. Twenty percent of the patients achieved a complete remission and were followed closely to determine its duration. The percentage of patients remaining in complete remission reached a plateau of 15% at 3 years, and these patients remained in remission for more than 10 years from the start of their FAC program.

If this could be considered a definition for *cure*, then it could be argued that effective chemotherapy such as FAC was able to cure 3% of metastatic breast cancer patients: 3% representing 15% of the 20% of patients who initially entered complete remission as a result of FAC. While this was very unimpressive, it was the first time cure could be reported as an outcome of chemotherapy for patients with stage IV breast cancer. It was only following Blumenschein's presentation of this data in 1983 at a conference in Scarpa, Italy that this encouraging fact was pointed out to him by Dr. John Mendelsohn, who was soon to be recruited as President of MDA.

Many interesting prognostic factors predictive of the outcome of patients with metastatic breast cancer also emerged from the very thorough and in-depth review of the 619 patients who first received FAC therapy. Of particular note was a research paper by Dr. Kenneth D. Swenerton, a medical oncology fellow from the Developmental Therapeutics Department. His assessment of the usual prognostic factors that were used to predict relapse-free survival and overall survival from the time that metastases were diagnosed included characteristics of the primary cancer such as tumor size, number of involved nodes, type of surgery on the primary, and prior chemotherapy. Surprisingly enough, these had no influence on the percentage of patients entering remission, the length of remission, or overall survival. Age, menstrual status, and disease-free interval from the initial diagnosis to the discovery of one or more metastases also had no significant effect on the response to FAC, the duration of any response, or the length of survival. However, decreased performance status and weight loss both had a negative correlation with response to FAC, as well as with duration of remission and survival.

The site of the metastatic lesions also had no significant effect on response or survival, although there was a higher remission rate in the small group of patients with only lymph node involvement. Patients with only bone metastases experienced a statistically significant prolongation of survival. But, if a patient with predominant bone metastases was found to have a metastasis in tissue other than bone, her remission rate and survival were no different from those with other metastatic sites.

Swenerton also evaluated the effect of tumor burden on response to FAC. He analyzed each patient with respect to tumor involvement in the 12 organ systems where breast metastases would most likely be found and scored each as zero, suspicious, minimal, moderate, or extensive. He assigned a semiquantitative numerical value to each score and summarized the values for each patient. The sites included breast, chest wall, lymph nodes, lung, pleura, liver, mediastinum, bone marrow, bone, and central nervous system. The numerical values for the score at each site were: 0 for zero, 1 for suspicious, 2 for minimal, 5 for moderate and 10 for extensive. Using this novel approach, Swenerton found a highly significant correlation between a patient's total tumor burden score and her response and survival following FAC therapy. This correlation was highest in the patients who achieved complete remission. Thus, 38% of patients with a small tumor burden (site summary score <5) achieved a complete remission, while 16% of those with a score of 6–12 entered complete remission, as did 8% with a burden of 13–20, and 7% with a score >20.

This was considered to be a remarkable observation which gave us a quantitative measure of tumor burden that could provide useful prognostic information. It also encouraged the increased use of surgical debulking prior to giving FAC in the hope that this would increase the likelihood of complete remission.

4.4 REFINING FAC

Around 1978, while the information about the effect of FAC and other Adriamycin combinations on metastatic breast cancer was still being collected at MDA, the dose and dose rate of these regimens was changed. For the first 3 days of each 21-day cycle, the Adriamycin dose was increased from 40 mg/m^2 to 50 mg/m^2 and was given by continuous IV infusion over 72 h. The intravenous dose of cyclophosphamide was increased to 500 mg/m^2 on day 1 and of 5-FU to 500 mg/m^2 on days 1 and 8. In addition, the dose rate was increased by compressing the treatment interval to 21 days. As long as a site of metastatic disease was responding, treatment was continued for a maximum of eight to nine cycles. However, it was decided that six courses would usually suffice for adjuvant therapy. This intensification of dose and dose rate was supported by observations that meaningful response to FAC decreased if there was a >20% reduction in drug dose or a treatment interval longer than 3 weeks. Thus, relatively early after its acquisition, a great deal of useful information was applied to optimize Adriamycin drug combinations, especially FAC, for the treatment of macroscopic and, therefore, microscopic metastatic breast cancer.

Dr. Freireich always stressed the value of clinical observation as a research tool. A relatively unimportant clinical observation about the use of Adriamycin with vinblastine, made during the time that the Medical Breast Service was exploring the effect of drug schedule on drug activity, is illustrative. Both drugs had been given separately to stage IV patients who had failed CMF chemotherapy. The response to continuous infusion vinblastine was 30% and to continuous infusion Adriamycin 60%. This level of response in patients previously treated with CMF caught the interest of Dr. Yap who wondered if a program that combined continuous infusions of vinblastine and Adriamycin might be useful if its activity were high enough. She reasoned that by starting with vinblastine on days 1 through 4 and following with rea-sonable doses of Adriamycin on days 5 and 6, she should expect at least a 55–65% chance of partial remission. The vinblastine was administered for 4 days, rather than only 1 day, before the Adriamycin in order to stall the cancer cells in mitosis, thus making more of them available for Adriamycin to kill as the vinblastine concentrations declined and cell division resumed.

The protocol was to be given to patients with metastatic breast cancer who had failed CMF. The first 20 patients did not respond as expected and there were only four partial remissions after 38 courses. Observing definite progression of disease following the initial course of the 20th patient, Blumenschein reversed the order of drug administration, giving Adriamycin on days 1 and 2 followed by vinblastine on days 3–6. The response was immediate and 29 additional patients were so treated. Sixteen achieved a partial remission, giving a 54% response rate. Later on, Dr. Yap came up with the explanation that when vinblastine was administered first, it was stored in body fat and released slowly into the circulation over the next 7 days, thereby persisting long enough to block Adriamycin activity when it was infused on days 5 and 6.

There are several questions regarding oncology that emerge from this vignette: (1) When does a protocol cease to be experimental? (2) Can there be an acceptable defense of departures from formal statistical analysis? (3) Can a clinical trial that is set up to answer a specific question provide other useful insights that were not anticipated in the original protocol? (4) Is it appropriate to enroll thousands of potentially curable patients in inferior therapeutic programs to prove an already obvious point?

The Adriamycin/vinblastine combination had modest activity as a front-line chemotherapy for patients with breast cancer. However, its 54% response rate, while respectable, was too low to make it a candidate program for consolidation treatment of microscopic metastatic breast cancer. Blumenschein felt that a consolidation adjuvant regimen had to have a higher response rate if it was going to contribute to a meaningful increase in the cure of microscopic metastatic breast disease. What he was looking for was a drug combination with a response rate of >70%.

None of the multitude of other adjuvant chemotherapy combinations had performed as well as FAC over the 10-years following its introduction in 1973. Every stage and subset of newly diagnosed breast cancer benefited from the addition of FAC adjuvant therapy. By 1988, data was available from 61 randomized trials involving over 28,000 women whose breast cancer had been treated with other adjuvant therapy combinations. These trials used chemotherapy programs that were not aggressive and for the most part were designed around CMF, CMFVP, L-PAM, and AC. At this time, 19% of the stage II, node-positive MDA patients treated with FAC and 41% of the randomized node-positive, stage II patients treated at other institutions with other adjuvant regimens had relapsed. Clearly, FAC remained the most efficacious drug program to spearhead the move toward cure of primary and metastatic breast cancer.

In 1987, Dr. Stephen E. Jones substantiated this impression when he reported a much-awaited comparison of outcomes between two CMF (Milan), one CMFVP (SWOG), one AC (Arizona), one L-PAM (SWOG), and the MDA FAC trials of adjuvant induction chemotherapy, using as a control a well-researched natural history database (NHDB) of stage II breast cancer patients who received only regional treatment. Whereas the L-PAM regimen had minimal effect on 5-year

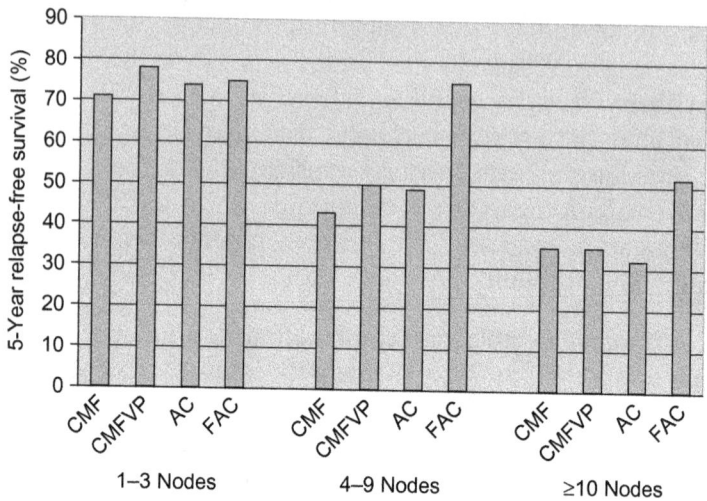

Figure 4.1 Comparison of 5-year relapse-free survival rates based on trials of different adjuvant chemotherapy regimens in stage II breast cancer patients (Data from Jones SE, et al. Am J Clin Oncol 1987;10:387–95).

relapse-free survival when compared to the NHDB results for regional therapy alone, the other adjuvant chemotherapy regimens all improved 5-year relapse-free and overall survival for patients with fewer than 10 positive lymph nodes. The 5-year relapse-free survival rates obtained with these regimens are shown in Figure 4.1 for the subsets of stage II breast cancer patients with 1–3 positive lymph nodes, 4–9 positive nodes, and ≥ 10 positive nodes.

There was little difference between these regimens in the 5-year relapse-free survival rate for the 1–3 node subsets, but FAC was clearly the superior regimen for patients with more extensive lymph node involvement. The results for FAC were particularly impressive in patients with ≥ 10 positive nodes as FAC was the only regimen that was shown in this group to be superior to regional therapy alone (5-year relapse-free survival: 52% FAC versus 28% NHDB, $P < 0.001$).

However, when Dr. Buzdar reviewed the results of the MDA FAC adjuvant trials for stage II and III breast cancer in 1990, it was apparent that there had been no significant adoption of the FAC program elsewhere in the United States. It was disappointing that the 1973 MDA outcomes remained a benchmark that had not yet been equaled in other clinical trials, many of which persisted in using Adriamycin as a single agent, limited the number of induction adjuvant courses to four, or eliminated 5-FU, without any apparent rationale. This nonrecognition of reproducible benefit was, to a large degree, due to the arbitrary rejection by most clinical investigators of clinical trials that lacked prospectively randomized controls. So these investigators were missing the opportunity to cure many patients with breast cancer, despite the fact that all the parts and pieces were lying about which would enable them to do so.

4.5 CISPLATIN LATE CONSOLIDATION

Late consolidation chemotherapy has to consist of a drug or drug combination with significant activity against Adriamycin-resistant or Adriamycin-exposed cancer cell clones. The strategy for its success in achieving a cure relies on administering the program to as small a residual tumor burden as possible. Skipper and Schable very clearly demonstrated in several animal tumor models, including breast cancer, that a sufficiently small tumor burden could be cured with chemotherapy. The set of prognostic factors associated with primary breast cancers predict that the doubling time for a rapidly growing tumor would enable it to grow in less than 3 years from a microscopic size to more than 1 billion cells, at which point chemotherapy would be unable to effect a cure. So the number of cells in a potentially curable tumor was of fundamental importance but was the great unknown. Fortunately, with the large number of breast cancer patients treated in a similar manner with a long follow-up, MDA physicians had the information with which to approach the answer and they estimated that chemotherapy had the potential to cure tumors only if they contained fewer than 1 million cells. This could be surmised by examining the break in the relapse-free survival curves of patients in complete remission who had been placed in a number of microscopic metastatic cancer substages, including stage IV, stage IV NED, IBC, stage III, and stage II $>10+$ nodes. Drs. Frei, Salmon, Goldie, and Coleman all have made similar estimates as to the size of a chemotherapy curable cancer.

The estimated tumor doubling time and location of the break in the relapse-free survival curve also provided a reasonable estimate that only 100,000 to 1 million cancer cells remained after effective adjuvant therapy. However, even these small cancers could evolve clones resistant to chemotherapy, so their eradication needed to occur before the second cycle of consolidation therapy. If a cancer is able to produce resistant clones after two cycles of consolidation therapy, the battle is lost. The strategy of employing a regimen of active, noncross-resistant combination chemotherapy immediately after induction adjuvant therapy evolved from this observation. This also is the major reason that it is necessary to seek out and test for drugs and drug combinations with a high level of noncross-resistance to other chemotherapy.

Cisplatin (CDDP) is one such drug. Blumenschein first encountered CDDP as a chemotherapy for metastatic breast cancer when verbal orders were misinterpreted and a 62-year-old woman received hepatic arterial CDDP instead of vinblastine for her widespread hepatic metastases. He read the riot act to anyone he could get his hands on and established a schedule to monitor the patient for any negative consequences. However, within 10 days her appetite had returned, the discomfort in the right upper quadrant of her abdomen had cleared, her liver had decreased in size. and her liver function tests had improved. It was obvious that she had very rapidly achieved a partial remission. This serendipitous event sparked Blumenschein's interest in CDDP because her primary cancer was aggressive, an advanced primary with 19 positive lymph nodes that was negative for ER and PR, as well as for the endothelial growth factor receptor HER2 (triple negative), and changed his thinking in regard to a potential role for this agent as part of a drug combination to be used after FAC as late consolidation chemotherapy.

Case Study

Joy

Stage IV NED as a Testing Ground for Adjuvant Therapy

Stage IV NED situations were another good testing ground for evaluating consolidation adjuvant drugs. Essentially, 100% of these patients have microscopic disease, so an increase in relapse-free survival is easily recognized. In this stage of breast cancer a single site of metastasis has been removed surgically or irradiated and the patient no longer has measurable metastatic cancer. But if nothing else is done, the occult sites grow and emerge, usually within 5 months. Usually, surgery eliminates any sites with $\geq 10^9$ cancer cells and radiation therapy can sterilize a focus of $\leq 10^7$ cells. However, these therapies are focused on specific anatomical regions. What oncologists need to obtain cures are effective drug combinations to clear the patient of any remaining sites containing $\leq 10^6$ cancer cells, regardless of their location.

Joy Barnes was 41 in January 1974, when she was diagnosed as having a T_2N_1 breast cancer. She underwent a modified radical mastectomy by a proficient surgeon in Jackson, Mississippi. The primary tumor was located in the upper inner quadrant of her left breast and two axillary nodes were positive for metastases. Joy received no further therapy.

A year later she began to notice discomfort on the left side of her neck. In April 1975, an isotope bone scan showed increased uptake of radioactivity in her fourth and fifth cervical vertebrae and X-rays confirmed the presence of lytic lesions in these vertebrae. She was referred to MDA for therapeutic recommendations and elected to remain in Houston for both chemotherapy and radiation therapy. Her staging studies showed no other sites to be suspicious for metastases. There was strong and compelling pressure to begin with radiation therapy to treat the obvious lesions in her cervical spine and avoid some catastrophic event such as a vertebral collapse that would compress her cervical spinal cord. However, this would delay the use of Adriamycin for over 2 months, enough time for microscopic metastases outside the radiation field to become clinically measurable and no longer capable of being successfully treated with chemotherapy.

It was unusual to find breast cancer patients with localized bone metastases and Blumenschein saw an opportunity to eradicate the microscopic lesions with FAC, while the bone response was monitored by the disappearance of pain and the appearance of blastic healing. Joy responded to FAC and her neck pain vanished after the first course of chemotherapy. This gave her physicians the confidence to continue the unconventional approach of beginning treatment with chemotherapy rather than radiation therapy. Upon completing the third course of FAC, there was blastic healing of the cervical spine lytic lesions. Blumenschein felt confident that Joy's cancer was responding, not only in her neck but also in her occult metastatic sites. Joy went on to receive 9 courses of FAC at 28-day intervals with a cumulative Adriamycin dose of 450 mg/m^2. She then proceeded with radiation therapy to her fourth and fifth cervical vertebrae, followed by an oophorectomy and consolidation therapy with CMF for 48 months.

Joy remains in unmaintained stable partial remission and in good health more than 35 years later. Technically, the fact that bone lesions undergo only blastic healing is what classifies Joy, as well as Janet, Carol and Lisa, as being in stable partial remission rather than complete remission. However, Blumenschein personally regards patients with stable partial remissions that have been maintained for more than 5 years as being in complete remission. He suspects that there may be something special about patients like Joy who have the cervical spine as a site for breast cancer metastases in that these patients have an unusually good prognosis and remissions of exceptionally long duration.

Case Study

Carol

Metastasis to Cervical Vertebra

Carol Rock was an informed and highly educated computer expert who was on assignment to the air force in Abilene, Texas. In the summer of 1988, at the age of 44, she developed a tender node in her right axilla. She saw her gynecologist, who confirmed the finding, gave her a prescription for an antibiotic, and told her to return in 3 days if there was no improvement. The node disappeared, but rapidly recurred within a week. She was referred for a mammogram on which a 2.5 cm mass was found in the tail of her right breast. She had an ultrasound-guided needle biopsy and the mass was diagnosed cancer.

Carol elected to have a quadrantectomy of the right breast with an axillary dissection. On August 10, 1988, the mass was removed. It measured $1.5 \, cm \times 0.8 \, cm$ and eight axillary nodes were involved with metastases. She was staged as having stage 2, T_1N_1 breast cancer, strongly positive for both ER and PR. Her surgeon was well trained, having recently completed a surgical oncology fellowship at Memorial Sloan Kettering in New York City. He had firsthand experience with what the finding of eight positive axillary nodes implied and, to his credit, guided her to the MDA program. At MDA, Carol received six courses of CAVe, underwent bilateral oophorectomy, completed 6 weeks of radiation therapy, and finished the therapeutic program with three courses of MCCFUD. When her assignment in Abilene was completed, Carol returned to her home base in El Paso. She did well, continued her computer work, and had follow-up examinations every 3 months. However, in June 1993, Carol was found to have a small stage 1, T_1N_0 cancer in her left breast. Again, she elected to have breast sparing surgery and was treated with lumpectomy and radiation therapy but received no adjuvant chemotherapy. This cancer was negative for both ER and PR.

In March 1996, Carol began to notice neck pain while driving her car. By June, this progressed to the point that it incapacitated her and she was referred to Dr. Howard Chang, a neurosurgeon in El Paso. Films showed almost complete destruction of the third cervical vertebra to the degree that her head was unstable. Dr. Chang felt that the only chance he had to prevent Carol from becoming severely paralyzed, or worse, was to remove the damaged bone and replace it with transplanted bone, which, hopefully, would regrow and give her cervical spine some structural integrity. In the interim, she would have to wear a cage-like device which rested on her shoulders and was attached to her skull with screws. She was told, "Life will be Hell for the next 6 months." Carol had no other option. So she went for it, thus living up to her pseudonym of Rock. The surgery was a technical success but the bone in her third cervical vertebra was found to be infiltrated with breast cancer. Fortunately, staging failed to show any other sites that were suspicious for metastases.

Radiation therapy could not be given to the area of healing bone. However, chemotherapy could be justified. So 2 weeks postoperative, he took the precaution of treating her with a little-used adjuvant drug combination: Adriamycin/vinblastine by continuous infusion every 21 days × 8, followed by FUMEP × 2.

Although, Carol has received a cumulative dose of Adriamycin that is more than 540 mg/m^2, she has had no clinical evidence of myocardial injury. She remains in good health, teaching computer science at the University of Texas, Austin, 20 years after being treated for breast cancer that had metastasized to her third cervical vertebra. We'll never know if this metastasis was from the original cancer or the second primary. But Blumenschein believes that she has passed the criteria necessary to be considered cured.

Case Study

Amy

Academia versus Efficacy

An exchange between Blumenschein and an "Ivy League" academician demonstrates the principles that each saw as unbreakable. They were consulting on a 28-year-old woman who 4 months postpartum was diagnosed with a T_1N_0 breast cancer 2 months after a mass was detected in her right breast. The cancer was triple negative (HER2-, ER-, and PR-). The patient chose preoperative chemotherapy and in August 2003 was started by her primary oncologist on AC $\times 4$ followed by Taxol $\times 4$ without the effect of this chemotherapy on her fertility having been discussed.

There was a measurable preoperative response to both AC and Taxol. However, a 0.7 cm focus of cancer remained in the breast after surgery and one node was positive on review of pathology. At this point, she self-referred to Blumenschein for a second opinion. With the advantage of the pathology report, Blumenschein pointed out that the axillary nodes seen on a mammogram obtained in August 2003 suggested that quite possibly the patient was T_3N_1 on starting adjuvant therapy and that this change in diagnosis would have made a different therapy program more appropriate for her. The prolonged interval from detection to starting 5 months of chemotherapy and the delay to late consolidation treatment were additional concerns. Yes, the patient was a candidate for breast radiation therapy but, before she began, Blumenschein suggested the way to insure the best possible outcome would be to repeat induction therapy with TAC $\times 4$, giving the Adriamycin by continuous infusion, followed by consolidation with 2 or 3 courses of FUMEP. Further action was then deferred until the patient could consider this recommendation.

The next day, the patient's father entered the fray. He asked to see a peer-reviewed paper supporting the need to return to chemotherapy after she had just completed a similar regimen. The need for literature support is a frequent weak point in the real world of clinical decision making. So Blumenschein knew his recommendation was sunk when he needed a publication to back it up. Real-world clinical decisions taken for a particular patient often cannot be defended by citing academic publications in which a randomized controlled clinical trial has been conducted in a group of patients who are exactly similar to the individual patient being considered.

The patient's Ivy League physician also vetoed Blumenschein's recommendation. At the time, it was considered unlikely that breast cancer recurrences would remain sensitive to Adriamycin, and there was a growing concern within the oncology community about limiting the cumulative Adriamycin dose in order to minimize cardiac toxicity. Furthermore, she had not heard of using complex chemotherapy combinations such as MCCFUD and FUMEP as consolidation regimens in the adjuvant therapy of breast cancer patients and would not consider their use unless there was a creditable randomized trial which demonstrated them to be safe and effective. She expressed very strong feelings about the need for physicians to practice "evidence-based medicine," and even questioned the need to give Adriamycin by continuous infusion.

Unfortunately, the patient's decision to stop systemic chemotherapy at this point probably lowered her chance of tumor eradication to less than 20%, whereas plunging ahead might have allowed a 50% chance of tumor eradication. A final blow was the rejection of Blumenschein's recommendation to give the patient Lupron[1] with each course of chemotherapy in an attempt to preserve ovarian function in a fertile 28-year-old woman who was receiving aggressive chemotherapy. In this case, Dr. Ivy League was aware of the concept and, in fact, her study group was evaluating its use in this situation in a randomized trial. However, Amy was not eligible to be included in the study, so she did not raise the issue with her or discuss the matter in any way.

Amy never regained her menstrual cycle, her cancer reappeared, and she was never cured. When Dr. Alfred DiStefano, who was one of Dr. Blumenschein's colleagues at both MDA and ACC, reviewed this case he made the following comment. "It is a shame to see someone so obviously intelligent and concerned for the welfare of her patients paralyzed into inaction and confined to the 'standard of care' by lack of the statistical anomaly of randomization. In my opinion this standard represents the 'average' at best and 'mediocre' at worst. Randomized trials are not needed to guide most of the things that we do every day. Experience and observation are still the prime tools of the art of medicine. Otherwise we could be replaced by assembly line robots!"

---

[1]Lupron is an LH/FSH inhibitor primarily used for treating men with metastatic prostate cancer. However, it also can minimize the gonadotoxic effects of chemotherapy by suppressing ovarian function while chemotherapy is being given.

CHAPTER 5

Marching Forward

In their independent review of the 619 patients with metastatic disease who were initially treated with FAC, both Swenerton and Legha noted the unusually favorable outcome in premenopausal women who had an oophorectomy within 6 weeks of initiating FAC. For some unexplained reasons, these patients had the lowest incidence of brain metastases, they experienced the longest remissions with a median duration of 33 months, and comprised the largest fraction of the 3% of patients who appear to have been cured by FAC. In the 1970s, Dr. Arthur W. Hoge, in Oklahoma, also reported that premenopausal women with stage IV breast cancer had a persistently increased remission rate when CMFVP was combined with bilateral oophorectomy and adrenalectomy. But the hormone therapy story was complex and probably governed by variable receptor sensitivity to hormones in different cancer cell clones. This resulted in a confusing situation in which a clone *in vitro* could not survive in the presence of estrogen, while it thrived with the hormone *in vivo*. The association between the low incidence of brain metastasis in premenopausal patients also is unexplained and requires further examination.

In immunosuppressed nude mice, estrogen-dependent tumors treated with the antiestrogen, tamoxifen, or deprived of estrogen had their proliferation suppressed, but there was no tumor regression or loss of cell viability. In some clinical trials, tamoxifen when given concurrently with chemotherapy seemed to have an additive effect on remission of ER+ cancers. Although this apparent effect did not reach statistical significance, this combination was associated with longer remissions and longer survivals than occurred in patients treated with cytotoxic chemotherapy alone. In particular, tamoxifen administered concomitantly with FAC tended to improve relapse-free survival and prolong overall survival in NSABP trials. These somewhat conflicting observations, together with Dr. Marc Lippman's 1978 report that ER+ breast cancers responded less well to cytotoxic chemotherapy, have introduced a note of caution about combining antiestrogens with chemotherapy. As a result, the majority of clinical trials avoid combining hormonal therapy with chemotherapy, save for oophorectomy in premenopausal patients.

There is one additional consideration related to hormonal therapy that pertains to premenopausal breast cancer patients: the older the premenopausal patient, the greater the likelihood that the chemotherapy will permanently impair her ovarian function. Of necessity, Blumenschein stumbled into the use of Lupron as a means of preserving fertility in a 35-year-old nulliparous breast cancer patient who needed chemotherapy but wanted to have children. She was given Lupron with each 3-week course of FAC × 6 and with each monthly course of MCCFUD × 3. It was a success, and the patient became pregnant 6 months following her third course of MCCFUD. Although not original with him, another favorite Freireich dictum emerged, "Necessity is the mother of great invention."

Subsequently, this approach was successful in preserving the fertility of at least three additional patients who were caught in this dilemma. When insurance companies objected to this use of Lupron, Blumenschein was able to find corroborating reports from Israel in which Lupron was used to protect fertility in young women who were treated with chemotherapy for Hodgkin's lymphoma. The only complication from Lupron, if it may be so termed, occurred when a 41-year-old unmarried attorney became pregnant following her last chemotherapy session but before the return of her menstrual cycle.

5.1 CALGB STUDY 8081

In the early 1980s, efforts began to conduct more clinically relevant chemotherapy trials. An example of such a trial was CALGB study 8081 that was sponsored by Cancer and Leukemia Group B, a clinical research cooperative that develops and monitors large interinstitutional trials. Patients with metastatic breast cancer were randomized to be treated either with CAF[1] or tamoxifen plus CAF in order to once and for all get a handle on the question of whether tamoxifen increased the

---

[1] It is characteristic of this field that CAF was really the same as the FAC regimen developed at MDA but was used by competitors who did not want to appear to be agreeing with us.

antitumor effect of CAF. Initially, eligibility was restricted to patients with metastases who had not received chemotherapy and to patients with metastatic disease who had not had adjuvant chemotherapy.

However, by the mid 1980s, the use of adjuvant chemotherapy for treating breast cancer was so common that it was difficult to find a relapsed patient who had not had prior chemotherapy. So it was becoming increasingly necessary for studies to include patients who previously had adjuvant drug treatment. Because cancer recurred in these patients after they had previously received adjuvant therapy, this raised the question of whether their relapse was due to the emergence of cancer cell clones that were drug resistant. In an effort to address this issue, 46 patients with advanced metastatic breast cancer who had received CMF adjuvant chemotherapy more than 6 months before, were added to the 379 patients already in the trial. The investigators concluded: "There was no difference in response rate, response duration, time to treatment failure, or survival between patients who had received prior adjuvant chemotherapy and those who had not. The addition of tamoxifen to CAF failed to enhance response rates or response duration in all the subgroups. Women who relapsed 6 months or more after completion of adjuvant chemotherapy did not have inherently drug-resistant tumors. They responded to standard CAF chemotherapy with the same response rate and survival as patients untreated previously with chemotherapy." Although several preliminary reports were released beginning in March 1983, this final analysis did not appear until February 1988.

CALGB 8081 put to rest any thought that tamoxifen might increase the activity of CAF. But it did not completely rule out the presence of a specific Adriamycin-resistant clone, as none of the 46 previously-treated patients had received CAF adjuvant therapy and Adriamycin had been administered at a low dose and a prolonged dose rate in the regimen that was used. Nevertheless, this was a worthwhile effort because it asked important questions about therapy of an important disease and required only a limited number of patients, time, and money. So patients were being used effectively to fathom the biology and the spectrum of drug sensitivity of the breast cancer cells.

The Breast Section of CALGB then stubbed its toe.

5.2 BACKSTEPPING ON FAC: FAC-LITE

For not entirely good reasons, the Breast Section of CALGB decided to conduct a dose—response study of FAC in which each treatment arm received the same total dose of each drug. Thus, the patients to be studied in CALBG 8541 had stage II breast cancer, status post mastectomy and were randomized to one of two treatment arms. In the first arm of the trial, patients received 5-FU at 600 mg/m^2 on days 1 and 8 and Cytoxan at 600 mg/m^2 and Adriamycin at 60 mg/m^2 on day 1 with a 28-day interval between courses. *Four* courses of this combination were administered to achieve a cumulative Adriamycin dose of 240 mg/m^2. The same drugs were used in the second arm of the trial, but were administered at a lower dose for each course: 5-FU, Cytoxan, and Adriamycin being given as 400 mg/m^2, 400 mg/m^2, and 40 mg/m^2, respectively. However, because the chemotherapy combination was administered 6 times with a 28-day schedule it resulted in the patients receiving the same cumulative dose of each drug. At the last minute, an issue arose concerning the already-accepted dose for CAF, so a third arm was created for CALBG 8541 in which the 5-FU and Cytoxan doses were reduced to 300 mg/m^2 and Adriamycin to 30 mg/m^2 at a 28-day interval for 6 courses, making the cumulative Adriamycin dose in this arm only 180 mg/m^2.

The question being asked in the two initial arms of the trial was: "Was the total dose received the significant therapeutic factor or was the dose per course of drug the determinant of therapeutic outcome?" While this issue had been addressed many times before and the answer was unequivocally established, it was not part of the CALGB's database. In retrospect, one wonders why there was any real need to read-dress this question when there were many more important issues, such as the combination of a taxane with Adriamycin and Cytoxan in an adjuvant program. The relapse-free survival and overall survival for the three arms evolved as expected. The most favorable response, as in the trial in stage IV patients that had already been conducted at MDA, occurred in the dose-dense arm in which patients received *four* courses of Adriamycin at a dose of 60 mg/m^2. Unfortunately, an upper limit of 240 mg/m^2 for total Adriamycin dosage had been arbitrarily established, so when this more effective Adriamycin dose was used, it could not be given for more than four courses. This arbitrary limit fixed for the future the number of courses of Adriamycin that could be given in a treatment program, despite the best efforts of Dr. Hortobagyi to bring some sense to the issue.

A second equally disturbing decision was made when the CALGB Breast Section violated the much-touted precept that decisions should be "evidence-based" and arbitrarily dropped 5-FU from CAF. Subsequently, these investigators took no notice of the fact that the response of their metastatic breast cancer patients to AC was poorer than that obtained with FAC $\times$ 6. AC $\times$ 4 now replaced the superior regimen of FAC $\times$ 6 and was locked in by several factors. It was easy, it eliminated 1 day of intravenous drug administration from each course, and there were fewer courses. Also there were fewer chemotherapy-related complications. Proponents of this inferior regimen defended it with the mantra that CALBG 8541 incorporated randomized controls, was conducted by noted investigators at prestigious cancer research institutions, and was accepted by insurance companies. Nowhere was the claim made that replacing FAC $\times$ 6 with AC $\times$ 4 improved cancer cell kill, an essential consideration that could eventually lead to *cure*. The underlying fault, of course, was that, as a less effective *induction* adjuvant program than FAC, it left more residual cancer cells for *consolidation* adjuvant therapy to clean up.

As a result of CALBG 8541, AC $\times$ 4 became the standard that was prescribed as the initial therapy for breast cancer patients with every stage of the disease. Subsequent trials made little or no attempt to incorporate readily available knowledge regarding a multitude of drugs, drug combinations, strategies, and breast cancer natural history information to actually bring about cures. Consequently, the general medical oncologist now was pressured to use an established, easy to remember, two-drug, insurance company-accepted chemotherapy for one of the more prevalent cancers in the United States.

In fact, the next significant move toward improving AC for induction adjuvant therapy was to evaluate the strategy of increasing the dose density of AC that was used for breast cancer adjuvant therapy. Unfortunately, this had limited application for most patients with metastatic disease because when they became study candidates they already had received a cumulative Adriamycin dose of 240 mg/m^2. This arbitrary upper dose limit reflected two common fears that were held by most oncologists. The first was that the tumor might at this point be resistant to Adriamycin. However, Adriamycin resistance seemed to be limited to cancers that had recurred while the patient was still receiving the drug or had recently completed treatment with it.

Once adjuvant AC had been adopted, with its four-course limit, it was unusual to experience a recurrence that was resistant to Adriamycin. Among other things, this strongly implied that four courses of AC were not sufficient to clear the Adriamycin-sensitive clones of cancer cells that were initially present.

The second fear was that heart muscle would be damaged when cumulative Adriamycin doses exceeded 240 mg. However, problems with myocardial damage that Blumenschein had experienced when Adriamycin was given by bolus intravenous injection disappeared after he used only a 72-h continuous infusion schedule. This infusion protocol also allowed repeat administration of a full 240 mg/m^2 Adriamycin dose. The reports from MDA by Legha, Benjamin, and Ewer were clear and have never been disputed. If they were not going to be accepted, what was the basis for their rejection? So the issue of heart muscle damage should have been put to rest in the late 1970s and early 1980s. Because the technique of continuous intravenous administration has not been generally adopted, Adriamycin continues to be used suboptimally and many patients have been deprived of the full benefits of adjuvant chemotherapy with this agent.

5.3 TAXANES REVISITED

When very high complete remission rates were reported in metastatic breast cancer patients who were treated with taxanes, Dr. Jean-Marc Nabholtz saw the opportunity to improve upon FAC as an induction adjuvant program for breast cancer. Through the Breast Cancer International Research Group (BCIRG), he organized and conducted the BCIRG-001 study to compare FAC to TAC (taxotere, Adriamycin, cyclophosphamide) for the adjuvant treatment of patients with operable, node-positive, breast cancer. The trial was conducted by 112 clinical investigators who enrolled 1491 patients in 20 countries between June 1997 and June 1999.

Results from this study were first reported in May 2002. At that time, the median follow-up of the patients on study was 33 months. The FAC and TAC cohorts were evenly matched as to number on study, median age, performance status, premenopausal status, mastectomy prior to chemotherapy, postchemotherapy radiotherapy, and postchemotherapy tamoxifen. Tumor stratification characteristics were one to three nodes and four or more positive nodes with 62% of the patients in each cohort in the one to three positive node subset. Approximately 20% of patients in the >3 node subset in each cohort had 10 or more positive nodes. The FAC dose was standard 500, 50, 500 mg/m^2, respectively, given intravenously every 21 days. The TAC program was closely matched as to dosage strength with taxotere 75 mg/m^2, Adriamycin 50 mg/m^2, and cyclophosphamide 500 mg/m^2 given intravenously every 21 days. Each 21-day course was administered six times.

This clinical trial was a model in its design, conduct, data collection, analysis, and evaluation. Relapse-free survival was greater with TAC in all nodal subgroups but most pronounced in patients with one to three positive axillary lymph nodes. In these patients, the risk of developing subsequent metastases was reduced by 50% and 90% of the one to three node-positive patients were disease free at 3 years, compared with only 79% of FAC-treated patients. However, it is possible that not enough adjuvant therapy had been given to patients with >3 positive nodes because only 69 and 67% of these patients were disease free in the TAC and FAC groups, respectively.

As the end of the twentieth century approached, despite the impressive results achieved with the use of TAC as induction adjuvant therapy, the great majority of clinical investigators studying the use of taxanes for adjuvant treatment of breast cancer were looking at its application as a late-consolidation adjuvant drug. The NSABP, CALGB, SWOG, and MDA all had used taxanes as a single agent for consolidation chemotherapy to be administered after mastectomy and four courses of AC adjuvant therapy. Response rates as high as 48% had been reported when taxanes were used as a single agent to treat metastatic breast cancer. But its efficacy was somewhat lowered when it was given following previous chemotherapy, with response rates ranging in the mid to low 30s.

In some clinical trials, adjuvant Taxol following AC × 4 did not benefit relapse-free or overall survival. As this was not the best use of an effective anticancer drug, it seemed appropriate to Blumenschein to keep searching for an efficacious regimen that, with no more than two courses, could complete the eradication of the small number of tumor cells remaining after the adjuvant application of such an effective induction program as TAC. It was clear that AC was not as effective as TAC and could not clear, or at least was less likely to clear, a microscopic residual focus of metastatic breast cancer cells. So by the mid 1990s, TAC should have replaced the ubiquitous use of AC ×4, which was beginning to be looked upon as the "penicillin" for treating breast cancer. It was difficult to see how any of the active programs were headed for the "home run" of cure if they persisted in ignoring certain facts:

1. AC ×4 was not as effective as FAC ×6 for achieving partial remissions when treating metastatic breast cancer (72% FAC vs. 62% AC).
2. TAC was far more effective in achieving partial remissions than FAC (93% TAC vs. 72% FAC).
3. Complete remissions were observed in up to 32% of TAC-treated patients.

Given that, when using FAC to treat patients with *measurable* metastases, Swenerton and Hortobagyi had made the impressive observation that the smaller the tumor burden, the higher the complete remission rate, then why should not the same logic apply to *microscopic* breast metastases? It seems reasonable that the fewer cancer cells that remain after surgery, radiation therapy, and induction adjuvant chemotherapy, the better will be the chance for an effective consolidation regimen to completely eradicate any remaining cancer.

5.4 THE DOSE-DENSE OPTION

By the early 1990s, it was evident that medicine had all the "bells and whistles," that if put together properly could cure most breast cancer patients who had a significant microscopic metastatic tumor burden. This would include stage II >3+ nodes, inflammatory breast cancer, stage II >10+ nodes, and stage III. A reasonable number of stage IV breast cancer patients also could be helped, such as stage IV NED, and those who had entered complete remission as a result of radiation therapy or chemotherapy.

Granulocyte colony stimulating factor (G-CSF) entered the marketplace in 1991 and made dose-dense therapy a further option. G-CSF is a hematopoietic growth factor that stimulates the bone marrow to generate granulocytes, a category of white blood cells that assist the body in managing infection. This permits chemotherapy to be administered at a higher dose rate, thus increasing its potential to increase tumor cell kill. The current term for this tactic is *dose-dense therapy*. In the late 1990s, the CALGB 9741 study tested this tactic in an adjuvant trial in 2005 patients with node-positive breast cancer who were enrolled in a randomized study that compared two similar programs:

1. Sequential: Adriamycin 60 mg/m^2, followed by cyclophosphamide 600 mg/m^2, followed by Taxol 175 mg/m^2.
2. Concurrent: Adriamycin 60 mg/m^2 together with cyclophosphamide 600 mg/m^2, followed by Taxol 175 mg/m^2.

Each arm received four courses of chemotherapy but was divided into two schedules, one to be given over 21 days per course, the other over 14 days. The 14-day program was considered dose dense. The 21-day program was our old friend AC $\times$ 4 followed by Taxol $\times$ 4.

All four treatment schedules were proven to be feasible and safe. However, at a median follow-up of 36 months, disease-free and overall survival were both statistically superior for the dose-dense arm with respect to both 3-year disease-free survival (85% vs. 81%, $P = 0.01$) and 3-year overall survival (92% vs. 90%, $P = 0.013$). G-CSF was given with each course of the 14-day treatments. In fact, it was the use of G-CSF, erythropoietin, antibiotics, and transfusions as necessary, that allowed physicians to push dose and dose rate more aggressively than in the past, thereby improving outcomes.

5.5 SLOW ADOPTION OF CONSOLIDATION THERAPY

What was missing? Blumenschein believed the available, but under-utilized, component in the pursuit of microscopic cancer eradication was an effective late-consolidation breast adjuvant regimen. Drs. James H. Goldie and Andrew J. Coldman at the Cancer Control Agency of British Columbia had speculated that to eliminate a residual tumor burden of 1 million or fewer cancer cells, the drug or drugs used would have to accomplish this with one or two treatments. Once the time had elapsed for a third round of treatment, they believed it was very likely that drug-resistant clones would have had sufficient time to appear. They reasoned that if this were the case, oncologists might want to begin looking at drug combinations containing mitomycin C such as FUMEP, in much the same way as they view radiation therapy. These combinations appeared to be promising candidates for a role in an intensive regimen for late-consolidation adjuvant therapy of an advanced stage cancer in complete remission.

Blumenschein's results from using MCCFUD and FUMEP in a limited schedule as a consolidating program in patients with IBC would appear to support this line of reasoning. MCCFUD was an attempt to increase the activity of CMF in patients who had relapsed after FAC or AC. In these patients, CDDP was given in a modest dose with methotrexate. The methotrexate was timed to have its greatest synergy with 5-FU and Cytoxan was delivered by continuous infusion over 72 h. Each cycle was 28 days apart. Three cycles were planned but only two were usually administered. In a population of breast cancer patients with a high rate of remission following FAC, CAVe, or TAC, such as patients with IBC, response rates were surprisingly high, with 75% having >50% tumor reduction, and MCCFUD was a welcomed consolidation adjuvant program. However, if the patients were initially Adriamycin refractory, response to MCCFUD was only 35%.

The use of MCCFUD for consolidation is probably the reason ACC'91 did so much better than MDA'94, which used 4 21-day cycles of Taxol as its consolidation regimen. In MDA'94, patients who relapsed following FAC, CAVe, or other adjuvant therapy, the response to Taxol was only 33%. Patients with IBC who received single-agent Taxol for late-consolidation adjuvant chemotherapy had a relapse-free survival rate of 49% at 3 years, whereas, as shown in Figure 3.1, if they received two or three courses of MCCFUD for the same purpose they had a 3-year relapse-free survival rate of 65% that was maintained for more than 10 years. Nevertheless, even the MDA Taxol consolidation program had a 35% rate of relapse-free survival that represented a significant gain when compared to the rest of the world's results in treating IBC.

5.6 THE IMPACT OF STATISTICAL DOGMATISM

The slow adoption of improved approaches to treating patients with breast cancer reflects the fact that this is an era that is dominated by statisticians who have been given the final say in interpreting the data being generated from the many clinical trials that are conducted in the United States and Europe. The accuracy of a new therapeutic observation, or the reproducibility of a modification in a longstanding therapeutic strategy, is only accepted after it has been confirmed by a repetition of the study with the subjects being randomized against an appropriate control group and with a difference in outcomes that can be reported with a statistically significant P value.

This statistical dogmatism creates a real-world dilemma for the oncologist and comes up against another Freireich dictum. He noted, "There is nothing more compelling than a cancer patient in need. That patient has come to her oncologist for help. She wishes to receive the best treatment; the treatment that in his or her judgment will give the best outcome." The patient does not come to be randomized. Drs. Freireich and Edward Gehan, a statistician at MDA, have provided a comprehensive review of this randomization issue in a paper entitled, "The Limitations of the Randomized Clinical Trial."[2]

Thus, the dilemma is, should the oncologist be a physician or an investigator? This dilemma has not been settled and becomes more difficult as more effective therapies are developed.

[2]Freireich EJ, Gehan EA. The limitations of the randomized clinical trial. Meth Cancer Res 1979;17:277–310.

Case Study

Beatta

Second-Guessing the System

In December 1999, Beatta Campos, a 37-year-old mother with three daughters, noted a mass in her right breast and consulted her physician. He reassured her that the mass was benign. However, the following May, the mass began to burn and she then sought the advice of Dr. Sanchez Basurto, a respected surgical oncologist in Mexico City. He advised her to have an immediate biopsy.

The needle biopsy showed a carcinoma. So on May 27, 2000, she had a modified right radical mastectomy. The breast contained a 4 cm × 3 cm × 2.5 cm, moderately well-differentiated infiltrating lobular carcinoma. Unfortunately, lymphatic permeation was present and 4 of 26 nodes from the right axilla contained tumor. The cancer was ER+, PR+, and HER2−. At this point, Dr. Basurto referred her to Blumenschein.

Beatta seemed to present a straightforward situation. Blumenschein proposed CAT × 6 induction adjuvant therapy, followed by irradiation and long-term tamoxifen. He reassured her that she should have a 90% chance of surviving at least 10 years with this program. He explained the need for an indwelling central venous catheter to be inserted during the CAT portion of her treatment so that she could be given Adriamycin by continuous infusion. He also mentioned that, at age 37, most women given these drugs have a high probability of entering menopause. If this did not occur spontaneously, it would be well to consider an oophorectomy soon after beginning tamoxifen.

Beatta had a great deal of concern about entering menopause because she had seen her grandmother suffer from severe depression when she entered menopause. In an effort to get her started on adjuvant chemotherapy, while keeping options open on ovarian function, Blumenschein added 7.5 mg of Lupron to the program with each course of CAT. She did well on this regimen. Although menstrual cycles ceased when she was given Lupron during her CAT program, they resumed when CAT was completed and Lupron could be discontinued. Her periods were regular and it was decided to follow her with more frequent observation. For some reasons, tamoxifen was never started.

Subsequently, Beatta remained under the care of a very competent medical oncologist, Dr. Raquel Gerson in Mexico and Blumenschein saw her infrequently. Almost 10 years to the date of her cancer diagnosis, he realized that she had never stopped her menstrual cycles and had not taken tamoxifen. The absence of recurrence after 10 years in a patient whose breast cancer was ER+, PR+ strongly suggests the CAT adjuvant therapy had successfully eliminated any residual tumor burden soon after it was started.

Beatta appears to have second-guessed the system and won. It was quite possibly time for Blumenschein to rethink his 10-year rule for designating complete remissions as cures.

Case Study

Lisa

The Patient of the Future

In August 2000, Lisa Bridges, age 43, was diagnosed with cancer in her left breast. The tumor was small and was located in the lower inner quadrant. She was treated with a modified radical mastectomy because three nodes from the left axilla contained metastases and there was extranodal extension into the perinodal fat with focal intravascular invasion. The tumor was ER−, PR−, and HER2+ with a 3+ score.

The following month, she consulted a medical oncologist in Evansville, IN who recommended that she receive adjuvant chemotherapy to be followed by radiation therapy to the peripheral lymphatics and the chest wall. An adjuvant therapy program was begun that month that consisted of the undeservedly popular AC × 4, followed by consolidation with Taxol as a single agent × 4. Fortunately, Adriamycin was administered by continuous infusion and the adjuvant program was completed without incident.

On a routine a follow-up examination in August 2002, a mass was discovered in Lisa's left upper lung. Lung tissue obtained by needle biopsy showed a poorly differentiated adenocarcinoma consistent with metastatic high-grade breast cancer. Several other sites were suspicious for metastases, including the hilum of the right lung and the 11th and 12th thoracic and 5th lumbar vertebrae. Lisa was started on weekly Herceptin (trastuzumab), a monoclonal antibody that blocks the HER2 receptor. Meanwhile, she visited MDA, Memorial Sloan-Kettering, Vanderbilt, and the University of Indiana. Each facility turned her down because they did not have an ongoing treatment protocol for which she was eligible.

In January 2003, Navelbine (vinoralbine), a vinca alkaloid that blocks dividing cells was added to her therapeutic regimen and Lisa first consulted Blumenschein later that month. His initial move was to refer her to Dr. Dan Meyer, a thoracic surgeon in Dallas, who was willing to attempt surgical removal of her lung metastasis. One week later, he operated and got her lung into a complete remission.

However, a major question was, how would resection of the lung lesion benefit a patient who had other sites of cancer spread? So Blumenschein used TAC × 6 for induction and FUMEP × 2 for consolidation adjuvant chemotherapy. Herceptin, which had been discontinued preoperatively, was restarted weekly with Navelbine, but had to be stopped after four doses because of declining cardiac function. Testing in the summer of 2003 showed blastic healing of the thoracic vertebrae and radiation oncologists proceeded with radiation therapy consolidation.

By September 2003, Lisa's hilar lymph nodes were becoming a problem and radiation therapy was called into action once again. Unfortunately, this resulted in radiation pneumonitis for which she had to receive steroid therapy. In July 2004, Lisa's pleura-based lesion returned. By November 2004, it had increased by 70% and a pleural nodule was surgically removed. Although this nodule showed no evidence of cancer, the surgery was repeated in January 2005 and cancer was present.

In November 2005, the lung lesion was again growing and Herceptin therapy was resumed. This time it was given with Abraxane, a formulation of paclitaxel bound to albumin. Seven months later, Lisa's chest scans had cleared and Abraxane was discontinued. Herceptin was continued every week until October 2006, when it again had to be stopped because of decreasing cardiac function. At that time, she was considered to be in complete remission. Herceptin was restarted when Lisa's cardiac function improved but had to be discontinued again in November 2007 when her cardiac function deteriorated again. At this time, restaging studies showed NED. Herceptin was resumed from January 2008 through July 2008 at which time the staging studies continued to show NED.

Lisa is going to require aggressive follow-up. By my dated criteria she may not be cured, but could be classified as in Herceptin-maintained complete remission in Abraxane complete remission or in Abraxane complete remission maintained by Herceptin. In this sense, Lisa Bridges is the patient of the future who never completely eradicates cancer clones but may control them with intermittent or continuous therapy. There is the possibility that the pattern of behavior demonstrated by Lisa's cancer will direct us toward a new strategy of maintenance therapy built around drugs like Herceptin that have specific targets.

CHAPTER 6

Concluding Thoughts — Where Do We Stand in the Quest for the Cure?

Where do we stand on achieving our goal: CURE in a reliable, repetitive fashion? What we have learned is that drugs are important in treating breast cancer and that combinations work better than single agents. There have been cures resulting from adjuvant chemotherapy since its introduction by Cooper. Bonadonna began treating microscopic breast cancer in the 1960s. Buzdar's introduction of Adriamycin in the MDA FAC program in 1973 materially improved the chance for a patient with microscopic disease to clear her body of cancer (Figure 6.1).

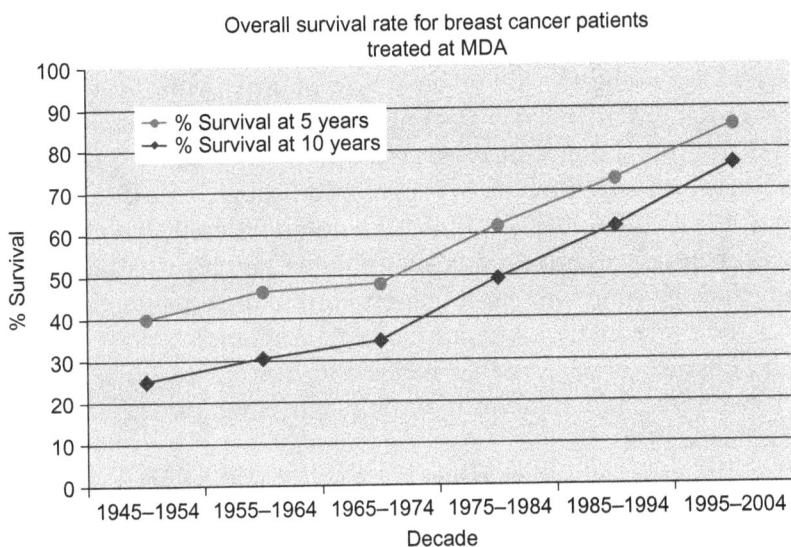

Overall survival rate for breast cancer patients treated at MDA

Figure 6.1 Based on Buzdar's data, the 10-year survival rate for patients with metastatic breast cancer has increased three-fold in the last six decades. However, survival did not increase significantly until Adriamycin was introduced as FAC adjuvant therapy (Data kindly provided by Aman Buzdar.)

Dr. Nabholtz is to be congratulated for his recognition of the superiority of TAC for induction and the need for it to replace FAC as induction adjuvant therapy.

There is a continuing need for improved consolidation adjuvant regimens in order to eradicate the microscopic tumor burden that remains after initial adjuvant therapy. CDDP, etoposide, and mitomycin C should be used in combinations, such as MCCFUD and FUMEP, only when other options have been proven less active.

There is a need for new drugs and combination chemotherapy regimens to be developed. Targeted molecular therapy is touted as the way of the future. At present, HER2+ patients have the option of using a very expensive drug regimen that incorporates Herceptin and Navelbine. However, will insurance companies be willing to pay for similar targeted therapies and, if not, will we be able to afford them?

6.1 CHEMOTHERAPEUTIC PRINCIPLES THAT HAVE EMERGED

- Future trials should be designed to emphasize tumor eradication and should not focus on questions that have already been answered.
- Multimodal regional therapy should be used as aggressively as possible. Decreasing the tumor burden in patients with metastatic cancer should improve chances of achieving a complete remission with TAC induction adjuvant programs.
- If a new drug program shows superior efficacy, don't let attachment to a previous favorite be an obstacle to adopting it. Recall the long delay before Adriamycin was incorporated into breast adjuvant therapy and the continued use of inappropriate or suboptimal combinations and schedules of Adriamycin (e.g., FAC-lite).
- The absence of measurable metastatic cancer creates a dilemma. Probably the best solution is to frequently monitor the patient and her tumor markers.
- Toxicity, especially irreversible damage, should be avoided if possible. The persistence of Adriamycin cardiac toxicity represents a major oversight on the part of medical oncology. Adriamycin should be given only by continuous infusion over 48–96 h. This necessitates placement of a permanent central venous catheter.
- Not all resistance that develops in some cancer clones is permanent, as evidenced the return of Adriamycin sensitivity in some cancers that initially became resistant to this drug.

6.2 PATIENTS HAVE AN IMPORTANT ROLE

Patient empowerment through education will play an increasingly important role in improving treatment outcomes. To that end, the following can be recommended:

- Do not hesitate to request a second opinion.
- A patient should ask her oncologist about the best route for cure. If the oncologist were in the patient's place, which treatment would they choose?
- Beware of waiting for a regimen or treatment to reach statistical significance in a clinical trial before accepting it if there is an intellectual pathway or compelling information to move ahead.
- Do not accept truncated or overly simplified regimens that may sacrifice therapeutic efficacy (e.g., FAC-lite).

Finally, it is important for everyone who is involved in the struggle against breast cancer to remember that the goal of treating breast cancer patients is cure. For the time being, all we know is that complete remission is the doorway to cure, and a prolonged complete remission usually is cure.

APPENDIX 1—MILESTONES IN ADJUVANT THERAPY

	1950s–2000
1950s	**Survival rate for stage IV breast cancer patients at MDA 1944–1954: 10.9% at 60 months, 3.3% at 120 months.** (Previously untreated, systemic metastatic disease.)
1957	NSABP (National Surgical Adjuvant Breast Program) formed. Howard E. Skipper and Frank M. Shabel, Jr. show breast cancer can be cured by chemotherapy.
1958	First adjuvant therapy clinical trial: Halstead radical mastectomy + perioperative ThioTEPA.
1960s	**Survival rate for stage IV breast cancer patients at MDA 1955–1964: 9.9% at 60 months, 4.0% at 120 months.**
1965	Roar Nissen-Meyer evaluates perioperative Cytoxan adjuvant therapy.
1966	Ezra M. Greenspan at Mount Sinai reports increased response to combination chemotherapy of advanced breast cancer.
1968	Bernard Fisher reports significant increase in 5-year survival of premenopausal patients with >4 positive nodes.
1969	Richard Cooper reports significant response in metastatic breast cancer from CMFVP. (ASCO abstract #57).
1970s	**Survival rate for stage IV breast cancer patients at MDA 1965–1974: 12.8% at 60 months, 4.7% at 120 months.**
1973	Gianni Bonadonna begins Milan CMF-12 adjuvant therapy trial; Blumenschein and Geoffrey Gottlieb write FAC protocol; MDA begins metastatic breast cancer trial.
1974	Aman Buzdar begins MDA adjuvant therapy trial with FAC.
1975	L-PAM NSABP trial in premenopausal patients; Stephen E. Jones and Sydney E. Salmon report adjuvant therapy with AC; CMF × 6 vs. CMF × 12 initiated by Bonadonna.
1976	NSABP moves to combination therapy with L-PAM and 5-FU; Milan CMF trial reported as positive for premenopausal patients with one to three positive nodes; FAC adjuvant therapy reported as positive by Buzdar as both pre- and postmenopausal patients with positive nodes have increased relapse-free survival.
1977	Buzdar, Blumenschein, and Gabriel Hortobagyi are criticized at meetings for being too aggressive and for using historical controls; NSABP moves to PMF, then to PFT and the breast oncology studies surge on; Bonadonna adds Adriamycin to CMF with CMFP+ AV.
1978	The East Coast, Midwest, and West Coast go with CMF; Texas and Arizona stay with Adriamycin.
1979	By this time, Adriamycin issues are clarified with respect to: (1) dose response, (2) dose rate, (3) timing with irradiation, (4) pathologic prognostic factors, (5) combination with hormone therapy, and (6) superiority to CMF questions answered with therapy of metastatic disease. Kenneth D. Swenerton's paper on prognostic factors is a cornerstone.
1980s	**Survival rate for stage IV breast cancer patients at MDA 1975–1984: 16.1% at 60 months, 7.4% at 120 months.**
1980	NSABP discovers Adriamycin. First consensus report: No adjuvant therapy indicated for stage I breast cancer; adjuvant therapy indicated for node positive premenopausal patients and perhaps for postmenopausal patients, if full dose used. FAC trial not recognized despite its superiority to CMF because its evaluation was based on historical controls.

1981	PAFT introduced for patients who had failed CMF; VATH reported by James Holland.
1982	Sewa Legha reports decreased cardiac toxicity of Adriamycin using continuous infusion schedule. Bonadonna reports significance of ER status and dose on CMF outcomes.
1983	Study of Adriamycin followed by CMF vs. CMF alternating with Adriamycin begun by Milan group.
1985	First meta-analysis; Second Consensus Conference: (1) established chemotherapy as standard of care for premenopausal patients with positive nodes. (2) Adjuvant therapy not generally recommended for premenopausal patients with negative nodes. (3) Tamoxifen recommended for postmenopausal patients with positive node and positive hormone receptor levels. (4) Chemotherapy may be considered but cannot be recommended as standard practice for postmenopausal patients with positive nodes and negative hormone receptor levels. (5) Routine adjuvant therapy not recommended for postmenopausal patients with negative nodes but may be considered in high risk patients.
1986	MDA reports improved relapse-free survival of stage II patients with non-cross-resistant drug combination consolidation therapy: MTX VLB following completion of FAC.
1987	NHDB (natural history database) and adjuvant therapy comparison study published by Jones. Dose–response relationship for Adriamycin in FAC clearly established using stage IV breast cancer patients.
1988	CALGB 8081 puts combined CAF+ tamoxifen to rest.
1990s	**Survival rate for stage IV breast cancer patients at MDA 1985–1994: 17.4% at 60 months, 11.2% at 120 months.**
1991	Arrival of Neupogen enables more intensive chemotherapeutic regimens. CALGB 8541 raises issues regarding significance of HER2 receptor in adjuvant therapy outcomes: (1) confirms plateau of Adriamycin efficacy at doses of 50–60 mg/m^2 in adjuvant patients, (2) suggests deintensification is not the same as intensification, (3) raises issue of studying dose–response relationships in adjuvant patients, (4) results misinterpreted with respect to optimum number of courses for Adriamycin adjuvant therapy.
1991	Demonstration that a chemotherapeutic program could or would not induce permanent drug resistance allowed reuse of Adriamycin to be considered if continuous infusion was used.
1992	Second meta-analysis of clinical trials.
1993	The drought of new chemotherapeutic agents is over with the introduction of Taxol followed by Navelbine, Taxotere, Gemzar (gemcitabine).
1995	The East Coast returns to single agent dose-dense sequential trials in the adjuvant setting without trials in stage IV breast cancer. Dose intense Adriamycin followed by Taxol followed by Cytoxan. NSABP shows no benefit from Cytoxan escalation. After the third meta-analysis, 5-FU vanishes from FAC and CAF.
1996	The efficacy of two non-cross-resistant adjuvant programs is established, but there is a continuing need for improved non-cross-resistant combinations.
1998	CALGB 9344: AC × 4 followed by T × 4 vs. AC × 4. At the 18-month follow-up, AC × 4 followed by T × 4 becomes the gold standard "penicillin" for breast cancer. Herceptin becomes available for HER2+ patients.
1999	Hortobagyi asks relevant questions regarding high-dose chemotherapy for breast cancer patients. High dose with autologous bone marrow transplantation is discredited. AC × 4 followed by Taxol × 4 sputters.
2000	Buzdar's MDA data remains reliable and becomes a standard.
2000s	**Survival rate for stage IV breast cancer patients at MDA 1995–2004: 36.0% at 60 months, 22.2% at 120 months.**

Stage I: Tumor <2 cm in diameter with no nodal involvement.

Stage II: Tumor <5 cm, >2 cm, with or without nodal involvement.

Stage III: Tumor >5 cm with or without nodal involvement.

Stage IV: Metastatic disease.

AC	Adriamycin, cyclophosphamide (Cytoxan)
ACC	Arlington Cancer Center (ACC'91 is a protocol I wrote here in 1991 for inflammatory breast cancer. In 1994, MDA started FAC-Taxol. These were the only protocols in which Adriamycin was given by continuous infusion.)
ASCO	American Society of Clinical Oncology
BCG	Bacille Calmette Guerin, a vaccine against tuberculosis that was used in cancer therapy as an immunostimulant.
BCIRG	Breast Cancer International Research Group
CAF	same as FAC (from people who wanted to do the same thing but didn't want to appear to be agreeing with us)
CALGB	Cancer and Leukemia Group B
CAT	cyclophosphamide, Adriamycin, Taxol
CAVe	cyclophosphamide, Adriamycin, etoposide
CDDP	cisplatin
CEA	carcinoembryonic antigen (a tumor biomarker)
CMF	cyclophosphamide, methotrexate, 5-fluorouracil
CMFVP	cyclophosphamide, methotrexate, 5-fluorouracil, vincristine, prednisone
ER	estrogen receptor: positive $+$, negative $-$
FAC	5-FU, Adriamycin, cyclophosphamide
FAC/BCG	5-fluorouracil, Adriamycin, cyclophosphamide/BCG
FUMEP	mitomycin C, cisplatin, 5-FU, etoposide (VP-16)
G-CSF	Neupogen, a white blood cell stimulant
HER2	an epithelial growth hormone receptor that is the gene product of the *HER2* gene (Herceptin is a humanized monoclonal antigen that blocks this receptor)
IBC	inflammatory breast cancer
L-PAM	L-phenylalanine mustard
PR	progesterone receptor: positive $+$, negative $-$
MCCFUD	methotrexate, cisplatin, 5-fluorouracil, cyclophosphamide, leucovorin (leucovorin rescues patients from methotrexate toxicity)
MDA	M.D. Anderson Cancer Center in Houston, TX
MOPP	Combination of Mustargen (mechlorethamine), Oncovin (vincristine), procarbazine, and prednisone used in the treatment of Hodgkin's disease.
MTX/VLB	methotrexate/Velban
NCI	National Cancer Institute
NED	no evidence of disease
NSABP	National Surgical Adjuvant Breast Program
SWOG	Southwest Oncology Group
TAC	Taxotere (docetaxel), Adriamycin, and cyclophosphamide
ThioTEPA	an alkylating chemotherapy agent related to nitrogen mustard